"In *Treating Psychosis*, Wright and her coauthors provide the reader with a treasure trove of cutting-edge cognitive behavioral therapy (CBT) techniques for treating psychosis—all in one succinct volume. Reflecting the evolution of CBT for psychosis over recent years, the authors outline a comprehensive treatment plan that will aid clinicians in making the best use of the myriad psychological strategies that have proven immensely helpful for individuals living with psychosis. The integrative model described in the book expertly links core CBT principles with the latest in mindfulness, acceptance, and compassion-focused strategies, producing an innovative new approach."

—**Brandon A. Gaudiano, PhD**, assistant professor at the
Warren Alpert Medical School of Brown University and
research psychologist at Butler Hospital in Providence, RI

"Building on both established cognitive behavioral research, practice, and treatment for psychosis and emerging work on acceptance-based and related approaches, the authors have put together a clear and highly practical therapist guide for the integrated treatment of psychosis. In addition to a comprehensive discussion of treatment processes and techniques, *Treating Psychosis* includes more than seventy pages of reproducible forms and handouts. This book is strongly recommended to anyone who treats psychotic disorders, either in groups or individually."

—**Martin M. Antony, PhD, ABPP**, professor of psychology
at Ryerson University and author of *The Shyness and Social
Anxiety Workbook*

TREATING PSYCHOSIS

A Clinician's Guide to Integrating
Acceptance & Commitment Therapy,
Compassion-Focused Therapy &
Mindfulness Approaches within the
Cognitive Behavioral Therapy Tradition

NICOLA P. WRIGHT, PHD, CPSYCH
DOUGLAS TURKINGTON, MD
OWEN P. KELLY, PHD, CPSYCH
DAVID DAVIES, PHD, CPSYCH
ANDREW M. JACOBS, PSYD, CPSYCH
JENNIFER HOPTON, MA

NEW HARBINGER PUBLICATIONS, INC.

Publisher's Note

"Emotion Regulation Systems" diagram from THE COMPASSIONATE MIND by Paul Gilbert, copyright © 2009 Paul Gilbert. Reprinted by permission of Constable & Robinson, Ltd.

"Form 4.1: Areas to Cover in Assessment" adapted from "Appendix C" in SCHIZOPHRENIA: THEORY, RESEARCH, AND THERAPY by Aaron T. Beck, Neil A. Rector, Neal Stolar, and Paul Grant, copyright © 2009 by The Guilford Press. Adapted by permission of The Guilford Press.

"Form 6.3: Strategies for Coping with Emotions," "Form 8.3: Behavioral Experiments for Distressing Thoughts or Delusions," "Form 9.5: Evidence for and Against Beliefs About the Content of Voices," "Form 9.6: Evidence for and Against Beliefs About the Cause or Origin of Voices," and "Form 9.9: Behavioral Experiment for Beliefs About Voices" modified from "Evaluating Beliefs About Voices" (p. 134), "Behavioural Experiments Form" (p. 139), and "Evaluating Coping Strategies" (p. 140) in THINK YOU'RE CRAZY? THINK AGAIN by Anthony P. Morrison, Julia Renton, Paul French, and Richard Bentall, copyright © 2008 Routledge / Taylor & Francis Group. Adapted with permission.

"Form 7.2: Activity Form" modified from "Activity Record" in C. W. Lejuez, D. R. Hopko, and S. D. Hopko. (2001). "A Brief Behavioral Activation Treatment for Depression: Treatment Manual." Behavior Modification 25(2):255–286. Copyright © 2001 Sage Publications, Inc. Adapted with permission.

"Form 8.2: Pie Chart for Alternative Explanations" and "Form 9.8: Pie Chart for Explanation of Voices" adapted from COGNITIVE THERAPY TECHNIQUES: A PRACTITIONER'S GUIDE by Robert L. Leahy, copyright © 2003 by The Guilford Press. Adapted by permission of The Guilford Press.

Distributed in Canada by Raincoast Books

Copyright © 2014 by Nicola P. Wright, Douglas Turkington, Owen P. Kelly, David R. T. Davies, Andrew M. Jacobs, and Jennifer Hopton
New Harbinger Publications, Inc.
5674 Shattuck Avenue
Oakland, CA 94609
www.newharbinger.com

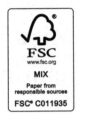 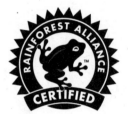

Cover design by Amy Shoup
Acquired by Tesilya Hanauer
Edited by Jean Blomquist
Indexed by James Minkin

Library of Congress Cataloging-in-Publication Data

Wright, Nicola P., author.
  Treating psychosis : a clinician's guide to integrating acceptance and commitment therapy, compassion-focused therapy, and mindfulness approaches within the cognitive behavioral therapy tradition / Nicola P. Wright, Owen Kelly, Douglas Turkington, David Davies, Andrew M. Jacobs, and Jennifer Hopton.
     p. ; cm.
  Includes bibliographical references and index.
  Summary: "Treating Psychosis is an evidence-based treatment manual for mental health professionals working with individuals who experience psychosis, a serious form of mental illness that causes delusions, hallucinations, and thought disorders. Psychosis is usually associated with schizophrenia, bipolar disorder, post-traumatic stress disorder, and severe depression. This is the first professional book to use a compassionate, mindful approach to treating psychosis using acceptance and commitment therapy (ACT) and compassion-focused therapy (CFT). The book provides clinicians with a pre-treatment overview and treatment implementation strategies, and focuses on developing a realistic action plan for treating patients with psychosis, as well as maintaining wellness"--Provided by publisher.
  ISBN 978-1-60882-407-6 (paperback : alk. paper) -- ISBN 978-1-60882-408-3 (PDF e-book) -- ISBN 978-1-60882-409-0 (ePub)
  I. Title.
  [DNLM: 1. Psychotic Disorders--therapy. 2. Acceptance and Commitment Therapy--methods. 3. Mindfulness. 4. Patient Care Planning. WM 200]
  RC489.C63
  616.89'1425--dc23
                          2014009368

Printed in the United States of America

16   15   14

10   9   8   7   6   5   4   3   2   1   First printing

To Dr. Aaron Beck, whose vision and approaches have changed countless lives.

Through his passion for understanding and working with those with psychosis, Dr. Beck has depathologized psychosis and made it possible for so many to pursue their goals and dreams as well as live fuller and more meaningful lives.

—The Authors

*

To my clients and those with lived experience of psychosis, who inspire me and have made my work and life so meaningful.

To my daughter, Emma, whose presence reminds me every day of the beauty and power of love.
To Dave, with love, for sharing part of the journey.

—NW

To my wife and family, who support me in all my travels, workshops, and writings.

—DT

To Natalie, Eliza, and Mariska, my family, my friends, and all my clients from whom I have learned so very much.

—OK

To Emma and Nic.

—DD

To the past, present, and future members of Yahara House.

—AJ

To R. A. H., in recognition of your struggles, successes, strength, and humanity. May you know peace. And to Guy, my love.

—JH

Contents

List of Figures

List of Forms

The following forms are available for download at http://www.newharbinger.com/24076. Please see the back of this book for instructions on how to access them.

Foreword

I am delighted to endorse this new guide for the treatment of schizophrenia. Since the pioneering work of Kingdon and Turkington (1994) in the early 1990s, cognitive behavioral therapy (CBT) has been developed into a powerful approach for promoting the recovery efforts of individuals with schizophrenia. The core theory of CBT for schizophrenia is supported by an extensive research base, and leads to strategies that drive interventions that promote positive and personally meaningful action as well as the removal of obstacles (voices, delusions, low energy) to goal-directed activity. The present volume provides a cornucopia of useful techniques that the CBT clinician can bring to bear to promote recovery of individuals with schizophrenia. Wright, Turkington, Kelly, Davies, Jacobs, and Hopton skillfully explain how values and committed action can be linked to core schemas and the generation of a problem list. I am pleased to see that the authors focus on compassion-focused techniques, which I have personally seen to be effective in promoting mastery over distressing experiences in many individuals with schizophrenia. They also describe mindfulness training as a useful approach to promote mastery while simultaneously helping to reduce anxiety. The authors deftly employ clinical vignettes to place the techniques in the setting of unique individual case formulations, which enhances understanding. Clinicians will find much here to incorporate into their CBT practices. The techniques can be used in individual and group settings. Both individuals with schizophrenia and caregivers will enthuse that the wellsprings of CBT have been strengthened with these new techniques to promote recovery.

—Aaron T. Beck

Acknowledgments

I would like to thank my clients who have shared their experiences with me. I feel honored to be able to be part of the journey with you. I would like to acknowledge the love, support, and inspiration of my family and friends as well as my colleagues and students in the Schizophrenia Program at the Royal Ottawa Mental Health Centre. Thanks to the many people at the Royal who have contributed to the vision of CBT treatment for those with psychosis. Thanks to Irit Sterner for the inaugural CBTp training together, Virginia Lafond for having the wisdom to bring CBTp to the Royal, Carlos Muira for having the vision to orchestrate the CBTp annual workshop series at the Royal, Tom Fogl for his passion for the well-being of his clients, Diane Hoffman-Lacombe and Raphaela Fleisher for their expertise and vision in bringing the group CBTp intervention to our forensic clients at the Royal, John Telner for the ABCs and the fun and laughter along the way, Leslie Sokol for her CBT training and for bringing me to the Beck Institute, the Turk for normalizing and inspiring, and Sarah Bertrim for her contributions to the original CBTp group manual. I would also like to extend a huge thanks to my beloved mother-in-law, Sandra Davies, and to Thomas Holmes, Megan Sawartsky, Will Hartley, Maria Harmaans, and Julia Grummisch for their editing. Julia was absolutely incredible in all of her professional assistance, including her creation of the treating psychosis website (http://www.treatingpsychosis .com). I would like to gratefully acknowledge Matthew McKay at New Harbinger for seeing the possibility of this work years and years ago and Randi McCabe for her generosity in sharing her proposal. My deep gratitude to Cathie Massel for her expertise through the CBTp manual development, and her ongoing support in so many profound ways. To my friends, thank you from the bottom of my heart for being like family through the joys and the pain. I would like to thank my Davies, Habib, and Wright families for their love and understanding when I was engrossed in the journey that has been this book. Finally, thank you to my parents, who inspired me through their sociopolitical values—I love you and miss you.

—NW

I would like to acknowledge all those service users and caregivers who have given me new insights into the nature of psychosis. The annual meeting of the International Conference of CBT for Psychosis has been a great encouragement. I would also like to acknowledge the ongoing cutting-edge input of Alison Brabban, Rob Dudley, Tony Morrison, and Sara Tai. Sara also contributed diagrams for the delusions chapter.

—DT

I would like to acknowledge and thank the many individuals who supported, supervised, and facilitated my clinical training, including Drs. Hymie Anisman, Michele Boivin, Kim Corace, Connie Dalton, David Davies, Sandy Drob, Hans DeGroot, Susan Farrell, Marilen Gerber, Anik Gosselin, Peter Henderson, Andrew Jacobs, Zul Merali, Amy Moustgaard, Daniella Sandre, John Telner, and Nicola Wright. It was a long road, but I learned so much from you all along the way—it has been well worth it.

—OK

I would like to thank the staff of the Anxiety Disorders Program at the Royal.

—DD

Thanks to my mentors and the clinical supervisors who have been pivotal in my training and thinking to date, particularly in the areas of trauma, psychosis, and severe mental illness. Special thanks to Drs. John Lyons, Jennifer Laforce, Susan Farrell, Nicola Wright, Marlene Best, Anik Gosselin, Geneviève Bouchard, Cecilia Taiana, Roy Salole, and to Mr. Joe Cassell.

—JH

*

Collectively, we wish to thank the University of Ottawa Institute of Mental Health Research, under the stewardship of Dr. Zul Merali, for the support and funding we have received. A special thanks to the clients and staff of the Schizophrenia Program of the Royal Ottawa Health Care Group. We wish to acknowledge and thank the University of Ottawa Medical Research Fund, funded by the Associates in Psychiatry at the Royal Ottawa Health Care Group, for the grants for the Group CBT for Psychosis study and the Voices Group study that served as part of the initial foundation of this book. Our thanks to the members of our two research teams and those involved in the implementation and evaluation of our CBTp protocols including Drs. John Telner, Sarah Bertrim, Alison Freeland, Tom Fogl, Ian Wienroth, Matthew Kerr, Verner Knott, Alain Labelle, Aleks Milosevic, Drew Kingston, and Diane Hoffman-Lacombe, Raphaela Fleisher, Susanna Konsztowicz, Carrie Robertson, Hayley Bowers, Dhrasti Shaw, Andrew Lumb, Krystelle Shaughnessy, Derek Handley, Julia Grummisch, and Ashley Beaudoin.

We wish to thank the wonderful staff at New Harbinger Publications including Tesilya Hanauer (for her incredible editing and understanding), Matthew McKay, Melissa Valentine, Jess Beebe, and

Amy Shoup. We would also like to thank Robin Walser for her feedback around ACT and Jean M. Blomquist for her diligent and insightful copy editing.

We would like to acknowledge the work of Drs. Aaron Beck, Judy Beck, Robert Leahy, David Kingdon, Paul Chadwick, Anthony Morrison, Andrew Gumley, Sara Tai, Alison Brabban, Paul Grant, Aaron Brinen, Neil Rector, Neil Stolar, Mark van der Gaag, Nicholas Tarrier, Richard Bentall, Steven Hayes, Patty Bach, Brandon Gaudiano, Kelly Wilson, Russ Harris, Paul Gilbert, Dennis Tirch, Chris Germer, Kristin Neff, Jon Kabat-Zinn, Zindel Segal, Lynette Monteiro, David Barlow, John Briere, Marsha Linehan, Martin Seligman, Rick Hanson, Derek Hopko, Carl Lejuez, Christopher Martell, and Neil Jacobson.

Finally, we would like to recognize the courage and resiliency of those with lived experience of psychosis. You inspire us, every day, to try to make a difference.

A Note About Integration and Application of Therapeutic Approaches and Language

Consistent with our approach to therapy and our clients, we have taken an individualized and flexible approach to the targeting of therapeutic strategies across therapeutic orientations that we have found to be helpful in working with those with lived experience of psychosis. As such, we hope this guide represents a clinically meaningful and empowering integration of approaches to benefit those with psychosis.

We have attempted to use the current most empowering and respectful language and terms in this book. We use the term "psychosis" instead of schizophrenia or schizophrenia-spectrum disorders, unless referring to research that uses the diagnostic terminology of schizophrenia. Consistent with a continuum-based model of understanding, we use the terms "distressing thoughts" and "delusions" interchangeably to speak to a range of culturally defined experiences and the way our clients think about and label their experiences. The term "psychotic experiences" is frequently used instead of psychotic symptoms in an attempt to use less pathologizing language that better reflects the experience of those with lived experience of psychosis. We realize that every experience of psychosis is unique, and, as such, we cannot do justice to the nuances around language that reflect the diversity in each individual's experience and environments. Ultimately, it is through a collaborative therapeutic relationship that we can discover the language that is most acceptable, respectful, and empowering for each individual.

Because this guide has been written for clinicians from diverse training and clinical backgrounds, we have attempted to make it accessible to clinicians with a range of knowledge and experience. Clinical information, material, and instructions may be repeated, at times, across chapters to reinforce principles but also to enable sessions, chapters, or modules to be implemented on a stand-alone basis, depending on the needs of the client and the setting (for example, inpatient stay, community-based treatment, and others). For therapeutic integrative purposes, we have used terms across a number of theoretical orientations (cognitive behavioral therapy, positive psychology, acceptance and commitment therapy, compassion-focused therapy, mindfulness, and behavioral activation). Rather than highlighting differences, we integrate these approaches by emphasizing common processes and therapeutic mechanisms. A glossary of clinical terms is provided on our website http://treatingpsychosis.com. A more integrative, humanistic, and empowering approach to psychosis based on evidence-based treatment strategies and clinical experience provides an extremely meaningful therapeutic approach for working with clients to enhance their ability to live to their fullest potential.

PART 1

PRETREATMENT OVERVIEW

CHAPTER 1

Introduction to Integrative Treatment for Psychosis

Cognitive behavioral therapy (CBT) is an effective treatment for a range of psychiatric and psychosocial difficulties including depression, anxiety disorders, substance abuse, eating disorders, and personality disorders. However, CBT for psychosis (CBTp) has historically received less attention, owing to the traditional reliance on pharmacological strategies for treating psychotic disorders. In parallel, there has often been an assumption that individuals affected by psychosis cannot benefit from psychotherapy. However, given that at least 50 percent of individuals diagnosed with schizophrenia experience persistent and distressing psychotic experiences despite adequate medication management and adherence (Robinson, Woerner, McMeniman, Mendelowitz, & Bilder, 2004), the need for additional treatment strategies is paramount.

This urgency for novel treatments is all the more pressing when the economic and social costs of psychotic disorders are considered. Although psychotic disorders affect less than 1 percent of the general population, in Canada schizophrenia alone accounts for an estimated CAD$1.12 billion in direct health care and non–health care costs (Canadian Psychiatric Association, 2005). Similarly, a recent review conducted in the UK concluded that the total cost per year of schizophrenia was £8.8 billion. Although less prevalent, costs for affective psychotic disorders were similar at £5.0 billion per year (Kirkbride & Jones, 2011). Finally, a US study examining costs of various chronic illnesses among a Medicaid dataset found that psychosis was the most costly chronic condition to treat per individual on an annual basis (Garis & Farmer, 2002). Costs to treat psychosis on a yearly basis exceeded costs associated with cardiovascular illness and diabetes. Importantly, psychosis was noted to be a contributing factor in approximately 70 percent of the most costly chronic illness co-occurrences. Economic costs aside, psychotic disorders are associated with significant morbidity and mortality and extensive disability in occupational, social, and day-to-day functioning as well as overall quality of life. Finally, though not often directly considered, the disability associated with psychotic disorders often requires that family members become involved in care. This involvement frequently strains the family's emotional and financial resources, leading to burnout and other negative impacts on quality of life and psychological well-being. Clearly, it is important to expand treatment approaches and maximize outcome, particularly with individuals persistently distressed by psychotic experiences.

Psychosis: Core Experiences and Features

Although many readers will already be familiar with psychosis and a range of psychotic disorders and their associated "symptoms," it is advantageous to describe the core experiences of psychosis as well as briefly outline those mental health problems characterized by psychotic features. Issues concerning the conceptualization, assessment, and treatment of specific issues related to psychosis will be discussed in depth in subsequent chapters.

Psychotic experiences, such as hallucinated voices and delusions in addition to difficulties with respect to thought, behavior, and emotion, can be observed transdiagnostically. *Delusions* are defined as erroneous beliefs that usually involve a misinterpretation of perceptions or experiences (in the *Diagnostic and Statistical Manual of Mental Disorders*, or *DSM–V*; American Psychiatric Association, 2013). As will be elaborated on in later chapters, while delusions can encompass a number of themes, the most frequently reported relate to notions of paranoia and/or persecution—for example, "the CIA is setting me up"—and reference, a belief that random events, objects, or behaviors of others are relevant to the individual. Other common delusions include those of a somatic, religious, or grandiose nature. Delusions are frequently, but not always, judged to be bizarre by the clinician. Care must be taken to evaluate a delusional belief in the context of an individual's cultural norms, practices, and beliefs. *Hallucination* is the clinical term to refer to the experience of sensory perceptions without a corresponding external stimulus (American Psychological Association, 2013). Hallucinations are most commonly experienced through the auditory system in the form of voices, but they can be experienced through any sensory modality including the visual, olfactory, gustatory, and tactile systems. Care must be taken to appropriately contextualize the experience reported by the individual, given that hallucinations can be a normative experience within some cultures. Moreover, as will be discussed below, hallucinations are broadly experienced by the population under a variety of circumstances.

While schizophrenia is the diagnosis most closely associated with symptoms of psychosis, symptoms of psychosis including delusions and hallucinations are a core feature of a number of different classifications including schizophreniform disorder, schizoaffective disorder, brief psychotic disorder, and delusional disorder. In addition, psychotic experiences can also be a primary feature of mood disorders such as bipolar disorder and, less frequently, major depressive disorder. Moreover, severe forms of post-traumatic stress disorder (PTSD), obsessive-compulsive disorder (OCD), body dysmorphic disorder, anorexia nervosa, hypochondriasis, and some personality disorders can present with psychotic features, particularly with respect to insight around the nature and severity of symptoms.

Conceptualization of Psychosis on a Continuum

Although traditional notions of psychosis reflect a decidedly categorical approach, consistent with the compassion-focused, value-driven approach of this treatment protocol, we, like others (Linscott & Van Os, 2010), propose that it may be advantageous to conceptualize psychosis along a continuum. This stance is born from the observation that, when looking at the clinical presentation of individuals with psychotic disorders, it is often the case that the core presenting symptoms reflect exacerbation of psychological, perceptual, or behavioral processes that were present long before the functional impact of these symptoms reached that of a diagnosable mental illness (Linscott & Van Os, 2010). In addition, psychosis-like experiences are prevalent among normative samples, free of serious mental illness (Linscott & Van Os, 2010).

Studies that have sought to determine the prevalence of hallucinations in both normative student samples and nonclinical adult populations have by and large found that a considerable proportion of individuals experience hallucinations at some point in their lives (Beck, Rector, Stolar, & Grant, 2009). For example, it is well documented that auditory, visual, and tactile hallucinations readily occur in healthy individuals during transition from awake and sleep-states and vice versa. In addition, mild sleep deprivation will evoke both auditory and visual hallucinations (Ali et al., 2011). Likewise, the experience of delusion-like ideas or beliefs appears to be fairly common. Notably, a recent review by Linscott & Van Os (2010) concluded that specific psychotic experiences including both delusions and hallucinations are three to 28 times more prevalent in the general population than schizophrenia itself.

Taken together, these data strongly suggest that psychotic experiences exist along a continuum, the presence of which does not automatically suggest or confer functional impairment or illness. Indeed, we suggest that psychotic experiences need only be addressed to the extent that they distress individuals and distract them from carrying out lives lived in the service of identified valued directions such as establishing and maintaining both platonic and romantic relationships, connecting with extended family, maintaining physical health, fostering volunteer work or paid employment, taking time for leisure and relaxation, or pursuing educational opportunities. In our experience, this stance toward psychotic experiences enhances clients' perceptions of safety in therapy, reduces stigma, and encourages their self-compassion and the forging of a strong therapeutic alliance. This is particularly important given the relatively high incidence of trauma experienced by this population (Schäfer & Fisher, 2011). Indeed, the negative reactions of others toward psychotic experiences as well as the self-stigma around the presence of psychotic experiences themselves often comprise a secondary form of trauma that greatly impedes clinical progress (Bendall, McGorry, & Krstev, 2006).

Suggested Target Audience and Format for Implementation

This treatment guide has been written for a variety of mental health professionals whose clinical practice frequently (or even only occasionally) requires practical knowledge of, and interventions related to, distress and disability associated with psychosis. As will be discussed below, multiple meta-analytic reviews support the implementation of CBT for psychosis on a one-to-one basis for individuals with ongoing distressing psychoses where treatment as usual, particularly neuroleptic medication, has been ineffective (National Institute of Health and Care Excellence [NICE], 2009). Many novel approaches implement group therapy, emphasizing, in addition to its cost effectiveness, the importance for participants to recognize that others experience similar problems as well as to feel less stigmatized, to experience the acceptance of other group members, and to improve social functioning. As such, the interventions described in this treatment guide have been designed in such a way that they may be used in both individual and group contexts. The sessions in the guide are written based on implementation in an individual therapy format. In chapter 3, we describe strategies for modifying the therapy sessions for group implementation as well as some special considerations for conducting therapy sessions in a group format. In addition, at the beginning of each treatment module we describe modifications for group implementation.

Implementation of Sessions

Clinicians can employ the guide in its entirety, progressing through each of the chapters in a linear fashion as clients grasp the relevant concepts and enhance their understanding and skills. This guide has been crafted in such a fashion that clinicians can also pull strategies, exercises, and tips for brief informal interventions with clients in outreach or assertive community treatment team settings as well as for those who have specific areas of distress. In addition, the treatment guide is designed so that sessions can be implemented in a "stand-alone" fashion. Thus, we have designed this guide to have the flexibility to be employed across a variety of settings, including: inpatient and outpatient settings in mental health facilities or units; community treatment teams and community settings; first episode psychosis teams; and forensic, correctional, and private practice settings (see chapter 11). Finally, though they are not the primary target audience of this guide, we hope that interested family members and caregivers of individuals distressed by psychotic experiences will be able to use this book to glean insight into the types of psychological treatments used with those who experience psychosis, and enhance their understanding of the factors that can trigger, exacerbate, and maintain distressing psychoses. This treatment guide can also be used by clients, family members, and caregivers to understand and reinforce therapeutic work.

Forms are provided in the appendix to enhance clients' understanding through psychoeducation and experiential skill–driven exercises. Ideally these forms or therapeutic strategies are first practiced collaboratively in session by the clinician and client. This way the clinician is able to reinforce effort, strengths, and progress as well as identify any misconceptions or difficulties that can be problem-solved in a collaborative and empowering manner. The exercises and information provided in the forms can then be used as a tool for clients to conduct between-session practice ("homework"). By taking this stepwise developmental approach, the aim is to appropriately individualize and target treatment with the goal of increasing experiences of success and mastery. Many of the forms in the appendix are available for download at the publisher's website for this book: http://www.newharbinger.com/24076. Also on the New Harbinger website, we have provided simplified versions of some of these forms. These simplified versions are provided to enhance individualization and targeting of treatment based on (1) stage of treatment and clients' development of therapeutic strategies and skills over the course of treatment, (2) stage of illness, and (3) cognitive function. Please see the back of this book for detailed instructions on how to access these forms.

In the interest of providing as accessible, up-to-date, and comprehensive clinical information as possible, we provide additional forms as well as information on research, assessment, treatment, and resources for the treatment of psychosis on our website at http://www.treatingpsychosis.com. We will update this website regularly. Issues that we could not address in this guide because of length and publication constraints will be covered on our website, as well as clinical materials, resources, and research that were not yet available at the time of publication.

Our ultimate goal in writing this guide is to enhance the quality of life of those who experience distressing psychosis. We believe our focus on more humanistic, process-oriented, and positive psychology approaches to recovery from psychosis illuminates a bright future focused on the strengths and potential of those who have lived experience with psychosis.

CHAPTER 2

Conceptual Model

In this chapter, we present the psychotherapeutic orientations and approaches that we incorporate into our integrated treatment model for psychosis. The rationale for this treatment model is explored with an emphasis on the functional connectivity between each of the approaches.

Cognitive Behavioral Therapy for Psychosis

The theory underlying *cognitive behavioral therapy* (CBT) is the notion that behavioral and emotional responses are strongly tied to the appraisal of events, which takes place in the form of cognitions (Beck, 1970). Stemming from this conceptualization, CBT seeks to address emotional difficulties using cognitive techniques as well as experiential, emotional, and behavioral approaches. Cognitive strategies within CBT aim to create awareness of distressing automatic thoughts and relevant cognitive distortions. Once this has been mastered, clients are encouraged to shift such thoughts with alternative explanations or possibilities (Beck, Rush, Shaw, & Emery, 1979). Later, dysfunctional belief systems—that is, *core beliefs*—and attitudes that flavor automatic thoughts can be evaluated (Beck et al., 1979). Experiential strategies aim to expose individuals to new circumstances in order to allow them to gather new information and insight into the validity of their perceptions. Finally, behavioral strategies aim to generate behaviors and skills that are effective in problem solving and will lead to broad changes in the way clients experience themselves and the world (Hofmann & Asmundson, 2008).

While cognitive behavioral therapy has been practiced clinically for over forty years, it is only recently that structured cognitive and behavioral interventions for psychosis have emerged. CBT for psychosis (CBTp) typically emphasizes fostering a strong, supportive, collaborative therapeutic alliance; providing psychoeducation and normalization; developing a cognitive behavioral conceptualization; developing skills or strategies to address stress, barriers, and distress related to experiences such as hallucinated voices or unusual beliefs; utilizing cognitive and behavioral techniques such as cognitive reappraisal and behavioral experiments to diminish the distress associated with positive symptoms; focusing on relapse prevention and recovery; and addressing secondary or comorbid problems such as substance use, anxiety, and depression (Kingdon & Turkington, 1994; Rector & Beck, 2002).

Similar to cognitive models of OCD (for example, Wells & Matthews, 1994), cognitive models of schizophrenia suggest that hallucinations and delusions occur when unusual experiences common to the majority of the population are misinterpreted and labeled as extreme, dangerous, or threatening (Morrison, 2001; Garety, Kuipers, Fowler, Freeman, & Bebbington, 2001). Resulting behaviors such as experiential avoidance serve to increase distress and negative mood states as well as to deny the individual the opportunity to gather disconfirming evidence. Indeed, as with other cognitive behavioral conceptualizations of psychopathology, the role of cognitive distortions, core beliefs, attentional biases, and experiential avoidance as well as safety behaviors are central to the development and maintenance of psychotic experiences (Tai & Turkington, 2009). Beliefs about the meaning and prognosis of a diagnosis of a psychotic disorder have also been identified as a clinical target in many cognitive behavioral interventions for psychosis (Tai & Turkington, 2009). In fact, normalizing unusual thoughts and perceptual experiences and emphasizing contributing external factors including psychosocial stressors has emerged as a central focus of CBTp to increase functioning and reduce stigma.

Positive Psychotherapy

Positive psychotherapy is an empirically validated, strengths-focused approach to therapy that emphasizes client strengths and positive emotions to enhance life meaning, well-being, and happiness (Seligman, 2002). Positive therapy approaches are implicit in the recovery movement for those with lived experience of psychosis (Copeland, 2010). The positive therapy approach is inherently empowering, destigmatizing, and affirming. Rather that focusing predominantly on symptoms, deficits, distressing emotions, and pathology, a positive psychology orientation incorporates strengths, qualities, resources, and an emphasis on the development of positive, pleasurable emotions to move in the direction of valued life goals and enhance meaning in life. In positive psychotherapy, strengths and positive emotions are crucial to engagement, a healthy therapeutic alliance, and a foundation and focus for treatment.

Acceptance and Commitment Therapy for Psychosis

Before discussing acceptance and commitment therapy (ACT), it may be helpful to briefly consider the broader context in which ACT has evolved. Studies examining the mechanism of exposure-based therapies have strongly suggested that the *function* of thoughts is far more important than their actual content (Barlow, 2002; Wells, 1994). Indeed, the successful integration of mindfulness techniques into clinical treatments such as Linehan's (1993) dialectical behavior therapy (DBT) and Segal, Williams, and Teasdale's (2002) mindfulness-based cognitive therapy (MBCT) suggest that the constructs of acceptance, awareness, and cognitive flexibility may have considerable utility in clinical practice. This "third wave" of behavioral and cognitive therapies is particularly sensitive to the context and functions of psychological phenomena and thus tends to emphasize contextual and experiential change strategies. For these reasons, third-wave therapies may be particularly applicable to the treatment of psychosis. CBT and acceptance- and mindfulness-based approaches have, at times, been assumed to be incongruent with respect to the goals of "control" and "change." However, in their integration these approaches can complement one another by emphasizing the understanding, exploration, observation, and acceptance of thoughts and feelings rather than the "stopping" and "controlling" of unwanted thoughts and feelings. In addition, although the ultimate goals of psychotherapeutic interventions for psychosis are many (including recovery, a reduction in distress, value-consistent living, working toward personal goals, and creating a more meaningful life), change occurs as a result of work toward these goals rather than as a goal in and of itself.

Central among these third-wave therapies is ACT (Hayes, Strosahl, & Wilson, 1999). From the perspective of ACT, mental health problems are thought to arise when the *process* of thinking is viewed as seamless with the *products* of thinking. Through the process of *cognitive fusion*, thoughts become functionally equivalent with actual events (Ciarrochi, Robb, & Godsell, 2005). For example, in an individual experiencing psychosis, the thought "I am being watched by the police" is evaluated not as simply a thought but rather as functionally equal to actual experiences reflecting the objective reality of being watched by law enforcement officials. Cognitive fusion is harmful in that it fosters avoidance of triggering aversive thoughts (Hayes, Wilson, Gifford, Follette, & Strosahl, 1996). Given that cognitive fusion facilitates both cognitive inflexibility and experiential avoidance that disrupts or impedes moving toward valued goals, ACT seeks to develop patients' psychological flexibility. At the center of this increased psychological flexibility are six core constructs and processes (Hayes et al., 1999):

1. Acceptance (rather than experiential avoidance)

2. Defusion (not cognitive fusion)

3. Contact with the present moment

4. Self-as-context or self-as-observer (instead of attachment to the conceptualized self)

5. Values (as opposed to not living consistently with values and/or pursuing avoidant values)

6. Committed action (in place of inaction, impulsivity, and persistence with avoidance)

Within ACT, values are the principle drivers behind action, acceptance, and defusion. *Values* are defined by Hayes, Luoma, Bond, Masuda, and Lillis (2006, p. 9) as "chosen qualities of purposive action that can never be obtained as an object but can be instantiated moment by moment." Values are not goals in that they are not things to be attained; rather, they are directions that can be lived out (Eifert & Forsyth, 2005). For example, while a goal might be "attend each of my child's soccer practices this summer," the associated value would be "being a good parent." It is important to note that interventions outlined in ACT are not ends in themselves; rather, they serve to promote living a life that is aligned with one's values. ACT promotes the practice of committed action to move the individual toward identified values (Hayes et al., 2006). Through committed action, the individual is able to build a larger and more flexible repertoire of psychological and behavioral responses (Hayes, 2004). Moreover, committed action serves to mitigate the suffering that can be a consequence of cognitive fusion and experiential avoidance. Thus, ACT is both a change- and an acceptance-oriented strategy. Hayes, Strosahl, and Wilson (2012) describe ACT as involving the processes of accepting, choosing, and acting, or engaging in committed action.

The evidence for ACT being effective in the treatment of psychosis, though limited at this point in time, is generally quite favorable. There is growing evidence that, among individuals affected by psychosis, ACT is effective in reducing the believability of psychotic experiences, reducing depressive symptoms, enhancing mindfulness, and lowering rates of rehospitalization and utilization of health services (Bach & Hayes, 2002; Bach, Hayes, & Gallop, 2012; Gaudiano & Herbert, 2006; Gaudiano, Herbert, & Hayes, 2010; White et al., 2011)

Compassion-Focused Therapy for Psychosis

Drawn from evolutionary social ranking theory, *compassion-focused therapy* (CFT) proposes that individuals with high levels of shame and self-criticism born from a history of abuse, neglect, or bullying often do poorly in therapy and are unable to feel safe and equal in their relationships with others (Gilbert, 1992; Gilbert, 2009). Importantly, shame and self-criticism evoke maladaptive patterns of thought and behavior that serve to maintain and exacerbate negative internal states such as psychosis (Gilbert et al., 2001). In the context of CFT, compassion reflects specific skills and attributes, the foremost being compassionate mind training (Gilbert, 2009). Specifically, *compassionate mind training* is a collection of techniques that facilitate the individual's increased awareness of negative interactions with the self. Over time, the blaming, self-critical stance toward oneself is substituted with an approach that emphasizes care for well-being, sensitivity, sympathy, distress tolerance, empathy, and nonjudgment (Gilbert, 2009). Compassion-focused therapy is based on the relationship among three types of emotion regulation systems, drive, safety, and threat. Using compassion-focused approaches enhances the safety or compassion-based soothing system while diminishing the threat-focused emotion regulation system and thereby enhancing the ability to activate (drive) and move in the direction of valued goals (see figure 2.1). Drawing upon techniques of many empirically supported psychotherapies, compassionate mind training is highly amenable to integration into emotion-focused therapy and CBT protocols.

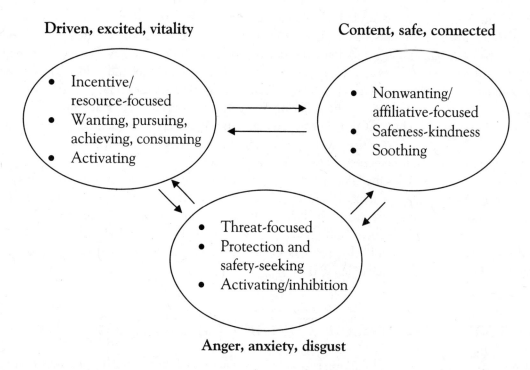

Driven, excited, vitality

- Incentive/ resource-focused
- Wanting, pursuing, achieving, consuming
- Activating

Content, safe, connected

- Nonwanting/ affiliative-focused
- Safeness-kindness
- Soothing

- Threat-focused
- Protection and safety-seeking
- Activating/inhibition

Anger, anxiety, disgust

FIGURE 2.1   Emotion Regulation Systems (Gilbert, 2009)

There is considerable prima facie evidence for the use of compassion-focused therapy in the treatment of psychosis. For example, it has been demonstrated that severity of illness in psychosis often correlates with the intensity of self-criticism and negative interpretations of the self, particularly in the context of complex presentations with comorbid mood and anxiety disorders (Tai & Turkington, 2009). Moreover, among individuals with psychotic disorders, self-criticism appears to herald a risk factor for relapse (Gumley, Birchwood, Fowler, & Gleeson, 2006). Finally, it has been suggested that the distressing hallucinated voices often experienced by individuals with psychosis tend to echo and perpetuate negative dynamics evident in the individual's everyday life with others (Tai & Turkington, 2009). Research and support for the effectiveness of compassionate mind training in the treatment of psychosis is growing. Laithwaite and colleagues (2009) found that among a small sample of individuals with psychosis who received a year-long intervention with integrated compassionate mind training, significant benefits were apparent with respect to measures of social comparison, mood, shame, self-esteem, and overall well-being. Braehler and colleagues (2013) found significant clinical improvements and significant increases in compassion. Notably, significant increases in compassion were associated with decreases in depression and social marginalization ratings. For a description of the application of group CFT for recovery after psychosis, see Braehler, Harper, and Gilbert (2013). For excellent resources on the science and practice of self-compassion, see Germer (2009) and Neff (2011).

Mindfulness for Psychosis

Mindfulness is a central and integral part of both ACT and CFT. Mindfulness has been incorporated in CBT as a CBT strategy and treatment approach (mindfulness-based cognitive therapy; Segal, Teasdale, & Williams, 2002; 2012). Mindfulness-based approaches have been applied to psychosis, with some modifications. Chadwick (2006) and Chadwick and colleagues (2005, 2009) have emphasized the implementation of mindfulness with those who experience psychosis. There is preliminary evidence that completion of mindfulness-based therapy is feasible for clients with psychosis and can positively impact overall psychological well-being and improve the ability to respond mindfully to stressful internal events (for example, Abba, Chadwick, & Stevenson, 2008; Chadwick, Newman-Taylor, & Abba, 2005; Chadwick, Hughes, Russell, Russell, & Dagnan, 2009; Langer, Cangas, & Serper, 2011; Langer, Cangas, Salcedo, & Fuentes, 2012).

According to Kabat-Zinn (2003), *mindfulness* can be defined as "the awareness that emerges through paying attention on purpose, in the present moment and nonjudgmentally, to the unfolding of experience moment to moment" (p. 145). The mindfulness process involves a nonjudgmental accepting of one's internal and external experiences. The process of coming into contact with distressing thoughts (or delusions) and feelings and experiences such as hallucinations and letting them pass without reacting to them enables exposure rather than the avoidance so often associated with "negative" or disturbing delusions and hallucinations. The decentered awareness in mindfulness facilitates the experience of cognitions as mental events in a broader context, and thereby facilitates a more metacognitive stance of decentering or defusing rather than getting "caught" in or reacting to thoughts or delusions, images, and hallucinated voices. The awareness and acceptance of thoughts, images, sounds, and/or hallucinated voices (positive or negative) diminishes the processes of judgment and self-criticism, including the internalized self-stigma that is so often present in those who experience psychosis. Present awareness provides an alternative process to the maladaptive processes of rumination and worry that so frequently accompany psychosis. As described in ACT, mindfulness-based approaches allow for a reduction in distress and an enhanced ability to engage in meaningful activities and the pursuit of valued goals (Harris, 2009).

A principal focus of mindfulness is to regard thoughts as "mental events" rather than accurate reflections of reality (Teasdale et al., 2000). Assuming this objective, detached stance toward thoughts is hypothesized to prevent the escalation of negative thought patterns that precede and follow deleterious psychological states such as psychosis (Teasdale, Segal, & Williams, 1995). It also allows clients to potentially foster a different relationship with these thoughts. This can be paramount in the context of psychosis, as symptoms and distressing beliefs may not abate with even aggressive pharmacological treatment.

Behavioral Activation for Psychosis

Behavioral activation (BA) is an empirically supported psychotherapy for the treatment of depression (Lejuez, Hopko, & Hopko, 2001). Although principles of BA have long been employed in the treatment of depression, these techniques were largely subsumed within general CBT protocols (for example, Beck et al. 1979). However, there has been increasing interest around stand-alone BA protocols, given that it has been demonstrated that BA is as effective as full cognitive therapy in treating depression both in the short (Jacboson, Dobson, Truax, & Addis, 1996) and long term (Gortner, Gollan, Dobson, & Jacobson, 1998). According to the BA model of depression, symptoms of depression persist because the individuals' predominant mood reduces their ability to both be exposed to and access reinforcement for nondepressed behavior while simultaneously reinforcing depressed behavior (Lejuez et al., 2001). Owing to this, BA seeks to increase exposure to the positive reinforcement that comes with engaging in healthy behaviors by providing a structured framework and rationale to reactivate behaviors, such as social interaction, that become largely dormant in depression. Ideally, as individuals become more activated in social and other domains, the reinforcement they receive increases, thus increasing the likelihood of further engagement in healthy behaviors at the expense of depressed behaviors. It is believed that this change in behavior will ultimately shift mood in a positive direction (Lejuez et al., 2001). Elements common to most BA protocols include psychoeducation around the influence of behavior on thoughts and emotions, identification of values and goals, mood and activity monitoring, activity scheduling, and graduated exposure to previously avoided activities.

It has been suggested that the negative symptoms of psychosis such as amotivation, alogia, and blunted affect reflect an attempt by the individual to moderate exposure to the consequence of positive symptoms, including the symptoms themselves, psychiatric treatment, and negative evaluations by others (Mairs, Lovell, Campbell, & Keeley, 2011). In addition, research indicates that negative symptoms are associated with defeatist beliefs about mastery and pleasure (Khoury & Lecomte, 2012). As in depression, this restriction of activity is strongly reinforced while simultaneously depriving the individual of the ability to access positive reinforcement for more value-driven behaviors (Mairs et al., 2011). Despite the suggested theoretical overlap between depression and negative symptoms of psychosis (for example, Hogg, 1996), there has been little investigation with respect to the efficacy of BA techniques in improving negative symptoms. In a pilot study by Mairs and colleagues (2011) employing a sample of eight individuals with negative symptoms of psychosis, it was found that treatment with a BA protocol was largely feasible and associated with reduced symptoms of depression and enhanced functional status. Importantly, treatment reduced negative symptoms while not evoking positive symptoms; however, these initial gains were maintained in only half of the participants at follow-up. While no firm conclusions can be drawn from this pilot study, the results align with the theoretical benefit that BA techniques may provide around activation and engagement in therapy and valued life goal attainment, thereby ameliorating negative symptoms of psychosis.

The Integrative CBT Treatment Model for Psychosis

The integrative treatment model for psychosis that serves as the foundation for our approach is presented in figure 2.2. The treatment model reflects a synthesis of elements of each of the interventions described above. The foundation and philosophy underlying our integrated treatment approach is based on positive psychology and recovery principles—that is, it is "positive psychology–infused." The core principle of this treatment guide is the importance of the client's identified values in driving shifts in thoughts, behaviors, and emotions with the ultimate goal of living a more meaningful and fulfilling life. Values are chosen directions in which an individual can always move no matter what specific goal is reached (Wilson & Sandoz, 2008). Flowing from this, we believe that it is helpful for clients to develop a mindful awareness of the present moment in order to allow the possibility of observing the function of emergent thoughts and/or behaviors relative to stated goals and, ultimately, values. This stance can foster cognitive flexibility, which helps clients to disengage from the struggle they are engaged in with distressing psychotic experiences. This struggle is often reflected by substance use as well as cognitive and/or experiential avoidance.

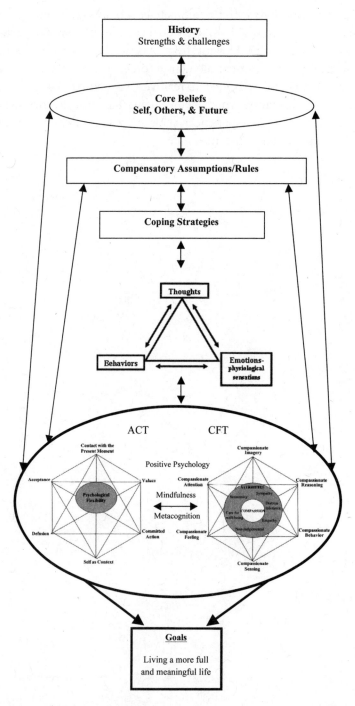

FIGURE 2.2   Integrated Treatment Model
(Elements adapted from Hayes, Strosahl, & Wilson, 1999; Gilbert, 2009; Beck, 2011; Tirch, Schoendorff, & Silberstein, in press.)

As the true function and meaning of our thoughts or actions are not always apparent, metacognitive and metaexperiential approaches are suggested as a means of facilitating clients' exploration of the meaning as well as the relative advantages and disadvantages of specific thoughts, feelings, or actions, both in the short and long term. Once the client, with the clinician, collaboratively identifies values, valued directions, and the actions needed to work toward valued goals, behavioral activation techniques can be used to consolidate committed action. Behavioral activation techniques, with their emphasis on values, can be integrated in a complementary fashion to collaboratively conceptualize and address the negative symptoms often associated with psychosis. In addition to identified goals and values, emphasis on the generation of compassion skills through compassionate mind training (CFT approaches) enhances the soothing/affiliation emotional system, thereby deactivating the threat emotional system that is frequently activated in psychosis. By developing and using compassion-focused strategies, clients are more able to link with their drive emotional system, thereby mobilizing committed action toward valued goals.

In addition, to enhance cognitive flexibility and reduce inaccurate perceptions of threat, CBT approaches employed in cognitive reappraisal and restructuring can be implemented to facilitate identification of possible cognitive distortions relating to the content, function, or meaning of symptoms (and other internal and external experiences) as well as alternative possibilities. Likewise, clients can be encouraged to undertake behavioral experiments in which evidence for the content, function, or meaning of a given symptom is gathered (if available) and weighed against alternative possibilities. The role of attention to threat and perceived threat in driving cognitive and experiential avoidance as well as causing, maintaining, and exacerbating psychotic experiences and anxiety is emphasized and addressed through self- and other-compassion skills.

In conclusion, we do not view symptom reduction as a primary (or necessary) goal of this treatment model. This integrated treatment model emphasizes clients forging a new relationship with their symptoms and experiences, the nature of which liberates psychological resources to pursue personal goals that embody tangible reflections of clients' values. Ultimately, this integrated treatment model aims to enable people who experience psychosis to enhance the quality and meaningfulness of their lives.

CHAPTER 3

Group Implementation

We have designed this clinician's guide to be used for both individual and group treatment. This chapter describes group implementation, including the rationale for group treatment, orientation and assessment, types of groups, criteria for selection and training of group leaders, group climate, and potential issues in group. Additional modifications for group implementation specific to each treatment module are provided in each treatment chapter.

Rationale for Group Treatment

The treatment sessions can be implemented in a group format in stand-alone sessions for inpatients and open groups, in modules, or as a complete group intervention. In our experience, group interventions can be experienced as extremely meaningful and therapeutic for clients with psychosis as the group format reduces isolation, increases normalization, augments hope, and provides opportunities to enhance social skills, social networks, and social support. In addition, the group format enables group members to learn from one another, receive reinforcement from peers, and benefit from positive peer pressure and support.

Selection and Appropriateness for Group

We recommend a group of five to nine individuals with two group leaders, although one group leader is possible depending on the group members' levels of wellness. We also recommend that group members have similar goals and foci for therapy and, if possible, that they are at a similar stage of illness (for example, first episode clients versus clients with longer term, more complex needs). Rather than focusing predominantly on client age, stage of illness is an important consideration when developing the group. For those with early phase psychosis or first episode psychosis, appropriate peer participants and those of a similar level of wellness are important. Please refer to the first episode literature for further information in this area (see the section "Early Psychosis/First Episode Psychosis" in the Resources).

Given the range in cognitive ability and cognitive flexibility, groups ideally should be targeted based on relatively similar levels of cognitive functioning. Material should be presented in multiple formats—written and oral as well as demonstration and role play. Repetition of concepts and strategies is essential. It is necessary to check frequently for understanding as well as to address fears and barriers to engagement and implementation of therapeutic strategies. Problem solving of any issues or predicted difficulties is essential, as is reinforcement of efforts and a focus on personal strengths and resources. Counterbalancing members based on level of motivation can be helpful, and gradual inclusion of more quiet members is advised due to social anxiety and potential fears regarding performance.

We typically run mixed gender groups with male and female coleaders. If there is a preponderance of one gender in a group, we discuss and process the gender demographics in the group. We prefer a minimum of two of each gender in each group. Same-sex groups can also be implemented to address gender-specific issues and concerns.

Pregroup Orientation Meeting and Assessment

We recommend individual pregroup meetings and assessments with one or both of the group leaders to discuss the group process and content, group and personal goals, and any concerns the prospective group member may have about participating in the group. We highly recommend beginning the values and goal clarification work and conceptualization in the pregroup assessment (see chapter 5 for more information). In the pregroup meeting, we also problem solve any potential barriers to group attendance or participation, modeling a problem-solving approach to issues or concerns that may arise. We discuss strategies clients would feel comfortable with group leaders using, such as strategies to increase participation and involvement. We also discuss their preferences as to how group leaders address elevated affect or distress in the group. Given the high level of comorbid substance use, we request nonuse of alcohol and other drugs before sessions and support a harm reduction approach rather than an abstinence-only model. By discussing potential issues proactively in the pregroup sessions and in the initial stages of group formation, group members experience ownership and buy into the process and strategies used.

Initial Group Session

Group guidelines are developed collaboratively by group members in the first session and emphasize confidentiality, respect, compassion, and a strengths-based focus. As part of this process, we also discuss how the group would like to address the potential situation of a member who becomes distressed or unable to participate in a session. Should a group member become extremely disorganized or acutely psychotic in session, the group has already discussed how this might be handled respectfully and caringly, and the group leader can intervene in an empathetic manner to address the client needs. If necessary, the group leader goes with the client to a quiet safe space (by a procedure based on previous group agreement on how these issues will be addressed). Fears and paranoia are handled in a caring, understanding, nonconfrontational, and nonchallenging manner to enhance a sense of safety in the group for later exploration of these themes. In our experience, group members typically find the group process to be an extremely helpful and normalizing therapeutic modality.

Type of Group

Groups can be conducted on an inpatient or an outpatient or community basis. Open groups are more suitable for inpatient clients, while closed groups can be beneficial to build on learning and to enhance safety, trust, and cohesion within the group. For open groups, session material is presented in a stand-alone format, often structured in rotating modules. Alternatively, in an open group, group members can generate the topic for the day based on previously prepared stand-alone session topics (for example, values, goal setting, coping with voices, assertiveness, and so on) or topics generated spontaneously by the group.

Following completion of closed groups, prearranged "booster sessions" for group members can be very beneficial. In addition, ongoing open groups can be offered that reinforce material that was covered in closed groups. In this approach, cross-fertilization occurs as participants who have completed closed groups participate in ongoing open groups, which bring together members from many previous groups. (This approach also addresses the need for a critical mass of group participants for holding open groups.) Participation in subsequent groups can be normalized and viewed as part of an ongoing process of staying well, just as exercise and diet changes require a sustained approach to be beneficial in the long term. Setbacks can also be experienced; using the term *tune-up* rather than "setback" or "relapse" can be experienced as more normative and less scary for clients.

Materials/Resources

Group seating arrangements are done to minimize an "us/them" atmosphere. Therefore, group leaders are interspersed with group members rather than placed apart in a classroom teaching style setup or as "expert" leaders separate from group participants. This setup of leaders among members implicitly acknowledges our common humanity.

Group materials can include a copy of the sessions and associated forms, a whiteboard or flip chart, and pens and paper for participants. Drinks and healthy snacks can enhance a social feel to the group as well as group attendance. A binder can be provided for each participant with new material added weekly. Group members can decide whether they wish to take their binder home each week or leave it with the group leaders and just take the forms and worksheets home. A binder with all session materials is given to each group member to take home when the group is completed. Group members can also be given a self-help book for CBT for psychosis (see Resources section).

Length, Frequency, and Breaks

Groups typically meet weekly and can range from forty-five minutes to two and a half hours. We typically conduct groups for ninety minutes without a break. Inpatient or open groups can be more frequent and of shorter duration. Material for each session should be stand-alone and not require development from previous sessions. We recommend a minimum of sixteen to twenty sessions for stand-alone closed groups. For clients with more complex needs and presentations, more than twenty sessions can be offered, depending on the functioning and goals of the group participants. Booster sessions, weekly sessions, or biweekly sessions in an open group format can also be offered after completion of the group sessions to reinforce benefits from the group and to enable practice and consolidation of skills.

Group Leaders

Group leaders should receive training in group therapy and as well as specific training for groups for psychosis. It is critical that clinical supervision be provided for group leaders who are relatively new to therapy for psychosis and/or group therapy. A coleadership model works well for risk, modeling, and coverage for absences. For training and supervision purposes, we typically have a seasoned group leader coleading with a more novice group leader. For some groups, we get each group member's consent prior to the first session to audiotape group sessions for clinical supervision and research purposes. In addition, we use these audiotapes for training purposes for students and professionals. Our clients typically find audiotaping nonintrusive; however, it goes without saying that, if consent is not readily given, we prioritize clinical need first and offer group services without taping. Content and process of each session should be discussed by leaders prior to the group and processed following each session.

Group Climate and Therapeutic Stance

The climate of the group should be warm, understanding, caring, and compassionate. These qualities should be modeled by group leaders and discussed as part of the group guidelines development process. The group should be strengths focused and reinforce effort and progress. The group climate influences group engagement, attendance, and cohesion.

Potential Issues

A number of potential issues can arise in group. These include overstimulation or activation of distressing affect, setbacks or decompensation, active distressing psychosis that can become upsetting or distressing to other group members, experience of voices or other hallucinations, disorganized speech or disordered thought that is difficult for group members to understand, disruptive behavior due to substance use, paranoid thoughts regarding group members or the group leader(s), sporadic attendance, poverty of speech and blunted affect, and minimal facial expressiveness. Offering social skills training, posing closed questions, cuing, providing a choice of responses, giving examples, targeting language level and content to the lower end of the group cognitive capacity, modeling by the group leader(s), and role-playing with the group leader(s) and in dyads or triads can be beneficial in addressing these issues. Having addressed potential issues or barriers, it is important to emphasize that feeling understood, sharing common experiences, developing social connections, and experiencing the support and reinforcement that come from the group process are extremely nourishing and empowering for many who experience psychosis. For more on potential issues that may arise in therapy, please see our website http://www.treatingpsychosis.com.

PART 2

TREATMENT MODULES

CHAPTER 4

Module 1: The Therapeutic Relationship, Engagement, and Assessment

This module is typically conducted in one to three sessions based on individualization for each client. Although the therapeutic relationship, engagement, and initial assessment are the focus for this module, therapeutic alliance building and the compassion-focused approach are ongoing throughout treatment. Areas to address in the assessment are presented in form 4.1 (see appendix). It is not necessarily therapeutically advisable to cover all areas in the initial assessment, as this may feel too overwhelming for clients. Just as the therapeutic alliance development is dynamic and ongoing so too is your understanding and assessment of your clients. Thus, the synergy of an understanding, compassionate, and strengths-based approach to relating to and assessing clients can, in and of itself, provide a corrective emotional experience and facilitate the development of a more hopeful and empowering narrative or personal story for clients.

Materials

See the appendix for forms. They are also available for download at http://www.newharbinger .com/24076. (See the back of this book for instructions on how to access them.)

Modifications for Group Implementation

The pregroup orientation and intial assessment should be completed individually by the clinician with each client prior to starting the group. Group process and typical group expectations are discussed in the pregroup assessment. Group process issues to highlight include a strengths-focused approach that incorporates psychoeducation. In addition, the importance of feedback and discussion between group leaders and group participants *as well as* among group participants is emphasized. We highlight the importance of a shared understanding and experience of issues and problems, normalization, and learning from one another.

As with individual therapy, let clients know that difficult affect may arise but that this is part of the important "work" of therapy. Encourage clients to attend group sessions even when they are having a "bad" day, as this is a key time to benefit from the group. Reinforce that clients will learn how to cope with difficult emotions in therapy and that other clients have found this kind of treatment to be helpful.

An example of group expectations can be given to each client as a handout, emphasizing the importance of confidentiality for trust and safety. To increase ownership and input, we typically generate group expectations collaboratively in the group. If any important areas are not addressed by the group members, these are introduced by leaders for group discussion.

Goals and Outline of Module (1 to 3 sessions, and ongoing)

This module focuses on therapeutic alliance, engagement, and assessment. Assessment is typically conducted in one to three sessions, but is by nature ongoing due to the dynamic nature of therapy, the alliance, and our clients' comfort and experience of self.

Overview of Treatment Area for Clinician

The chapter should be reviewed, by you, as clinician, prior to the session. The review should include any content that is important to cover in the initial history and assessment as well as pertinent psychometric and paper-and-pencil assessment measures (see form 4.1). Additional information on assessment and assessment measures can be found in the Resources section or on the companion website http://www.treatingpsychosis.com.

Check-In

The initial sessions are essential for establishing a warm and safe therapeutic environment for clients. Complete a client check-in, including current well-being, reason for the referral for therapy services, and an exploration of client attitudes toward (potentially) commencing treatment with you. To enhance engagement, provide an understanding and overview of what will be covered in the initial interview and assessment. Provide an overview of, and the rationale for, the assessment process, and answer any questions. When completing the assessment and any assessment measures, inform clients of who will have access to this information and any limits to confidentiality. A written consent with limits to confidentiality can be used. If appropriate, ask clients to complete paper-and-pencil measures. (See our website http://www.treatingpsychosis.com for a list of measures.) Remember to tailor the way you present information about the assessment and treatment process to the level of wellness and cognitive functioning of your clients. Assessment measures can be experienced as intrusive and/or overwhelming, and may increase paranoid or suspicions thoughts. Pacing, breaks, and clarification of any misunderstanding of questions are key to engagement and receiving quality clinical information for therapy purposes. Always start this and every other check-in with emphasis on a strengths-focused approach; be sure to ask clients about their strengths, accomplishments, positive emotions, personal qualities, and more, as appropriate.

Clinician Stance

Your stance should be one of warmth, caring, normalization, and validation during the initial engagement and history-taking process. It can be helpful to let clients know that even if they have told their story many times, it is important for you personally to hear about their experiences so you can understand and get to know them better and be of the most help to them. You might ask, "Are you willing to share your story again with me so I can get to know you better?" or say, "Please humor me. I know you have probably answered these questions many times, but I want to hear it from you." The personal history or narrative is a crucial part of the therapeutic engagement and therapy process. It is also an important opportunity to provide validation, understanding, support, and hope. In addition, it is an opportunity to highlight existing strengths, resources, and coping strategies as well as previous problem solving, coping, and efforts by your clients. Consider using an approach that incorporates a positive introduction of self by clients to highlight the strengths-focused approach to your assessment and treatment. Consistent with an ACT approach, it is important for you, as clinician, to try strategies that you will be asking your clients to do and to try engaging in mindfulness and compassionate mind training in your own life. In addition, the therapeutic values of compassion and a strengths orientation entailed in this approach to therapy should be embodied in your therapeutic stance with your client—and with yourself as therapist!

Therapeutic Engagement and Assessment Process

The Critical Role of Engagement and Rapport

The stance within the therapeutic relationship is premised on a strengths-based empowering approach that involves radical collaboration between the clinician and client. The key qualities of the therapeutic alliance are warmth, empathy, caring, genuineness, positive regard, and active involvement of the client. Taken together these therapeutic qualities can be framed as compassionate. That is, the model that we propose for working with those who experience psychosis not only has compassion as its foundation, but it also incorporates the synergy of the modeling of compassion and the development of compassion for self and others. According to the Dalai Lama, this compassionate stance involves not only sensitivity to the suffering of others (and the self) but also a profound commitment to attempting to relieve pain or suffering (which we address through, among other things, compassion, values, and valued life goals). Therefore, the therapeutic stance in our model encompasses the sensitivity to suffering and the motivation or commitment to address and relieve it.

As Gilbert (2010) points out, this approach to the therapeutic relationship, process, and goals is based on the evolutionary neurophysiology of reassurance, safety, caring, and attachment. This compassionate approach to therapy and self is critical in working with psychosis, given the high rates of trauma history and the trauma that can be experienced as a result of psychosis. In some cases, the treatment of psychosis itself can be traumatizing (for example, being brought into treatment involuntarily by the police). As Gilbert (2010) indicates, compassion affects brain functioning and emotion regulation in positive ways, while Greenberg and colleagues (1993) emphasizes the ideal therapeutic relationship is, in and of itself, an emotion regulator.

The empowering, strengths-focused, and empathetic therapeutic stance and process is consistent with Chadwick's (2006) emphasis on "radical" collaboration in the therapeutic relationship. In addition, the ACT conceptualization of the therapeutic relationship of clinician and client as fellow travelers on the journey of life is consistent with both a recovery approach and Kingdon and Turkington's (1991, 1994, and 2005) normalizing approach. These approaches, as well as CBT, conceptualize psychotic experiences on a continuum with "normal" experience rather than as dichotomous entities or experiences. A normalizing approach, including the cotraveler metaphor, is implicitly humanistic, destigmatizing, and depathologizing. This understanding of the therapeutic relationship enables the client (and clinician) to experience a greater sense of connectedness. In our model, the therapeutic relationship is oriented toward wellness versus illness and strengths versus symptoms or pathology, and it emphasizes recovery, values, and pursuit of valued life goals. Given the often extremely isolating nature of the experience of psychosis, an approach that has at its core the appreciation of the ubiquity of suffering and our common humanity is connecting. The ACT focus on the importance of the pursuit of a meaningful and fulfilling life is appealing from a recovery perspective. Similar to positive psychology and recovery-based models, the therapy focuses on enhancing what is strong, not "fixing" what is wrong.

The importance of the therapeutic relationship (and clinician competence) in engagement, assessment, and treatment in integrative therapy for psychosis cannot be overstated. There tends to be a misconception that the therapeutic relationship is not as central in cognitive behavioral therapy as some other therapeutic orientations. In addition, the importance of the experience of affect and therapeutic work with emotions—in cognitive behavioral therapy in general and in cognitive behavioral therapy for psychosis in particular—has often been greatly minimized. Our integrated treatment approach highlights the importance of the therapeutic relationship. Our model emphasizes the exploration, experience, regulation, and expression of affect and a deep and sophisticated understanding of the experience of psychosis rather than a superficial attempt at "challenging and eradicating" the client's symptoms. The model focuses on the process and function of thoughts and behaviors. For example, what purposes do worry, rumination, and attention to threat serve, and what are the client's beliefs regarding the pros and cons of each?

The therapeutic alliance and goals are based on the client's values and valued goals in therapy that are synergistic with the overarching model (and the clinician's values). One of the enhancements brought by these approaches is the increased focus on the integration of values and one's experience of self and relationships in the therapeutic work. In addition, the therapeutic approaches are used by both the client and the clinician (for example, the clinician engages in mindfulness practice and incorporates a mindful approach to self and the client in the therapeutic relationship) (Siegel, 2010). A beautiful synergy emerges as the therapeutic relationship is implicitly, in and of itself, an empowering and emotion-regulating relationship within which the client is able to strive for optimal well-being.

Special Considerations in Working with Psychosis

A number of issues can come up in therapeutic work with those who experience psychosis. Clients can be hesitant to discuss thoughts, beliefs, and voices due to therapeutic safety concerns. We cannot overstate this: trust and safety are paramount and essential to meaningful and adaptive therapeutic work in this integrated CBT treatment approach to psychosis. Previous invalidating experiences when clients have talked about unusual thoughts, experiences, or voices can contribute to a lack of safety in discussing experiences. In addition, a perceived stigma by others as well as self-stigma related to the diagnosis of "schizophrenia" or hearing voices can act as a barrier to disclosure and therapeutic work. The perceived potential for increases in medication or length of stay when unusual thoughts or experiences are reported to health care providers can impact on the client's willingness to work on certain issues or topics in therapy. Limits to what the clinician will disclose to the treatment team should be discussed with the client at the beginning of treatment, and any client concerns addressed proactively and transparently. Rapport, safety, understanding, and validation are critical foundations for the therapy work.

Individualizing treatment is critical, and adjustment of therapy to address any increase in symptoms should be made to enhance safety and trust. The client is given the ability to drive the pace in the therapeutic work. Instead of working directly with symptoms like voice identity, content, relationship, and so on, therapeutic work on identifying values and goals as well as the core beliefs (such as those underlying low self-worth) that drive the theme and content of the symptoms are addressed. The focus of the therapeutic work on core beliefs and schemas undermines the core beliefs supporting the content and believability of distressing symptoms. In addition, the "symptoms" can serve other purposes, such as a compensatory purpose (for example, making the person feel special or important) or that of staving off loneliness. Therefore, it is essential to explore what purpose symptoms may serve for the client. If isolation or loneliness is an issue, activity scheduling, including social activities, can be developed with the client. If a sense of worthiness and value is an issue, coping strategies, self-esteem-enhancing strategies, and value-driven goals can be an initial and ongoing focus. A focus on valued goals can redirect energies from the client's preoccupation with symptoms to more strengths-focused and meaningful pursuits. Exploring the advantages and disadvantages of the amount of time and energy spent on symptoms using motivational interviewing strategies can help the client to engage in more meaningful goal-directed activity or committed action. In summary, a compassionate therapeutic approach to the lived experience of clients is fundamental. The therapeutic stance is one of respect, compassion, understanding, and normalization. Through this therapeutic stance, the client experiences validation and safety in the therapeutic relationship and is able to work toward meaningful life goals.

The Critical Role of the Therapeutic Relationship

Now we'd like to shift for a moment from the theoretical to the experiential. Dr. Wright provides the clinical example below to illustrate the critical role of the therapeutic relationship.

One of my clients perceptively describes the importance of the therapeutic relationship in the compassion-focused integrated CBT treatment approach for psychosis this way: "You saved my life. When I first came into therapy, I felt so unsafe and alone. My delusions and my beliefs about my voices were like a solid block of cheese, dense and impenetrable, but now they are like Swiss cheese; we have blown holes all through them. Because of our work together, the beliefs don't hold true and haunt me in the way they used to. During tough times, I hit on the solid parts, [distressing inaccurate beliefs], but from what I have learned in therapy with you, I can blow holes right through them again—and I do."

Every Christmas I get a pack of Life Savers from this client, and every year I remind her that she saved herself and continues to do so.

On a similar note, every day as I walk into work I pass people from all walks of life who are struggling with, and trying to work through, what can feel like the demons of psychosis. Through a safe and compassionate therapeutic relationship, they are able to search for and find meaning, live a more value-consistent life, and work toward their valued goals. Every day as I walk past them and hear my name called, I know that the work we do together matters, that the relationship we share is sacred, and that the therapeutic journey we travel together is connecting and leads to a more enriched experience of self and life for both of us.

As described above, the therapeutic relationship is the thread we use to tie together the therapeutic tapestry of empathy, understanding, meaning, and connection. Without this secure, caring, and empowering therapeutic base, progress toward valued goals is more limited, and the therapeutic impact of feeling heard and understood in a strengths-oriented manner is diminished.

Engagement and Therapeutic Goals

The therapeutic goals in working with psychosis are typically reducing distress, enhancing understanding and acceptance, and increasing quality of life so clients can be freer to focus on valued goals and directions. Client goals are pursued by collaboratively identifying and constructing values and valued life goals. The pursuit of meaningful goals inherently involves clients' acceptance of their lived experience and/or symptoms, as well as clinicians' working with them to help them to be open to experiencing symptoms as they pursue their valued goals. Given that clients who have lived experience of psychosis have often experienced invalidating responses by others and/or stigma associated with their symptoms or diagnosis, it is important that you welcome and explicitly support the discussion of distressing thoughts and unusual experiences in an understanding and empathetic manner. A stance of gentle curiosity and respect is a corrective experience in and of itself, as this stance is implicitly normalizing, destigmatizing, and validating.

Our Values and Views as Clinicians

As clinicians, the importance of exploring our thoughts, beliefs, and attitudes toward mental health issues and our clients has often been underemphasized. ACT emphasizes not only the values of the client but also the values of the clinician. As such, our understanding of the lived experience of others and our values are critical in the therapeutic work that we do. Below we provide an exercise to help consider our common humanity in the path that can lead to psychosis.

—EXERCISE: A Path to Psychosis

Imagine that this is your life story:

You experience a serious complication at birth, or you do not meet important developmental milestones early in life because of extreme neglect or physical and sexual abuse. Your classmates bully you at school, or you have a family member who is predisposed to psychosis. In your teen years, you begin to smoke weed to deal with your past and some of your feelings. You feel down, alone, and not good enough. Given your past, you begin to feel like people are out to get you.

You begin to withdraw as you feel more fearful. You try to make sense of "unusual" perceptions and physical sensations. As you try to make sense of these experiences, you are hypervigilant and attend more and more selectively to threat. You misinterpret some of your perceptions or experiences.

You pay attention only to information that fits with your fears. You begin to isolate yourself more and more because you sense—and fear—that something is really wrong with you and those around you. Your isolation cuts you off from the possibility of learning a different way of looking at your life and experiencing yourself and others.

Finally, you decide you will take a "risk" and you tell a close friend or family member—someone you think it's safe to talk to—about what you've been thinking and experiencing. Instead of "getting" what you have to say, he says he's worried about you and needs to take you to the hospital for your own good.

You say, "No, I'm okay," and you withdraw more. Then, one terrifying night, the police break down your door and take you to the hospital against your will. They say you are at risk of harming yourself. You're terrified. You lose your possessions—and your rights. You're told you have something called schizophrenia—an illness often associated with hopelessness and stigma. You're watched all the time—they call it "1:1 observation." They take away your cigarettes…and you go into withdrawal.

You start to hear a voice threatening you. You're scared, and you start screaming and running. Someone calls, "Code white! Code white!" All the hospital staff come running at you, a needle jabs you, and you're out cold.…

Slowly, groggily you wake up…when?…where? The world crashes in. You're restrained physically and chemically. They offer ECT—"It's in your best interest," they say.

After getting out of the hospital, you begin to lose contact with friends and family. You lose your dreams, your hopes, your job, and you aren't able to return to school. You live in poverty, in substandard housing where you're not safe.

Finally, one day after years of different health care providers who seem to come and go, you find someone who actually listens to you and seems to care, someone who wants to hear your story, someone who understands you and reminds you of qualities and strengths you forgot that you had.

Finally, you start on the journey of rediscovering who you are and what you want to do in this life. You start on this journey with a clinician who hears you and "gets" you…and you begin to move into your future life with hope.

It is our gift as clinicians to go on that journey together with our clients, to help them discover meaning, hope, and a future.

Special Considerations in Engagement

At times in the therapeutic relationship or over the course of the therapy sessions, you may be incorporated into your client's thoughts, voices, or delusional beliefs or system. Voices may comment on therapy or your intentions, abilities, or personal qualities. Your clinical judgment is important here; it is possible to express explicitly at the beginning of therapy the importance of transparency and bidirectional feedback in the therapeutic relationship. As with any cognitive behavioral therapy work, feedback (both positive and constructive or negative) should be requested at the beginning and end of the session, as well as periodically during each session and across multiple sessions.

Sample Comments and Questions

Therapeutic comments and questions such as those listed below can be used to enhance the therapeutic alliance. A collaborative therapeutic style involves welcoming client feedback and input at the beginning of session, throughout the session, and at the end of each session. Comments and questions such as these can be modified to suit your client, the therapeutic relationship, and your therapeutic style. (See our website http://www.treatingpsychosis.com for a more comprehensive list of sample questions that can be used to elicit feedback from clients as well as sample Socratic questions.)

- As I said before, this therapy is for *you*. You are a partner and active participant in the therapy process. As we explore your experience, I encourage you to let me know at any time if you have questions or concerns. For example, please let me know if your voices say anything that you feel might get in the way of therapy or of you experiencing a safe therapeutic relationship with me.

- As we talked about in the past, I will check in regularly to ask you for feedback on how the therapy or session is going for you. As I do with all my clients, I will check in to see whether you have experienced any changes in the content or quality of your thoughts and/or voices in the therapeutic relationship with me.

- Do you think there might be anything that could get in the way of you and me talking openly about both positive and (potentially) distressing experiences in therapy? If so, what could we do in advance to solve that problem?

- Do you think that you would be able to let me know if you feel anxious or fearful (or if voices are active) in the therapy session? What about if your fear, paranoia, or voices are getting in the way of our discussions and work in session? If you don't feel comfortable letting me know and cannot let me know why, what could I or we do differently for you to be able to express these thoughts or feelings to me?

- What has been helpful and not so helpful in the session today?

- Did you experience any fearful, paranoid, or unusual thoughts in our session today?

- Did you hear any voices in session today?

- Was there anything in our discussion that did not fit for you (about unusual thoughts, beliefs, voices, and so on)? Was there anything that bothered you in what I said during the session today (or in past sessions)? Please let me know at any time.

- What do you think your voices think and/or feel about me? Do your voices ever comment (in a negative or positive way) about our therapy or about me as a clinician? If so, let's try to talk about that so we can work together toward your goals.

Of course, when, how, and to what degree these types of questions are posed in therapy is a clinical judgment based on your evaluation of your clients' sense of safety, trust, and readiness, as well as their understanding of their psychotic experiences, including their relationship with their voices. Too much focus on possible responses of the voices can engender suspicion, giving clients the mistaken impression that you, as the clinician, know more than you are saying. Clearly, it is a sophisticated and clinically individualized dance we do to be present with clients in a way that creates a safe environment for the therapy experience. Of course, we as clinicians cannot purport to be the experts on our clients' experiences, but we can try to do a delicate and graceful dance in exploring and seeking to understand distressing experiences, even as we intertwine that dance with judicious psychoeducation.

Given the often-fluctuating nature of psychoses, any and/or all of the above issues can be dynamic; they can change and evolve through the course of therapy. It is important for you and your clients to be aware of the tendency for psychotic symptoms to be exacerbated during times of stress and experiences of vulnerability. Again, it is important to problem-solve in advance what might help clients, based on coping skills they've developed as well as previous experience. Soliciting input from clients about what you can do to help eases anticipatory concerns and enhances their experience of you as client centered, understanding, and empowering.

Another issue that may come up in the therapy that impacts therapeutic rapport is active voices during the session that are distracting and/or demeaning to clients or you. Again, proactively agreeing on the best way to deal with this possibility can enhance client efficacy and engagement. For example, an agreed-upon hand gesture by your client to slow the pace, discontinue the session, or explore the experience of the voices in session can be extremely helpful. Your acknowledgment and understanding of the difficulty in focusing and engaging at these times is beneficial.

As in any type of therapy, symptoms such as paranoia or voices may actually increase initially and/or at different times during the therapy process. Therefore, it is important to indicate to your clients proactively that symptoms (and distressing affect) can increase at times in therapy. Together you can then collaboratively problem-solve how an increase in symptoms can be dealt with, thereby reducing premature termination or concerns regarding the benefits of therapy. In addition, work done at the beginning of therapy on enhancement and development of coping skills and emotion regulation strategies can be emphasized and reinforced by the clinician (see chapter 6).

Strategies such as a stop hand sign or "panic button" are respectful and empowering. Through these types of strategies, your clients have control over the pace at which assessment and therapy are conducted, the ability to take a break or disengage at any time, and the agency to reengage when ready. This client-driven approach not only applies to the frequency, length, and content of the sessions but also to how much clients share and at what pace. The experience in therapy of having a sense of control in the session speaks to the issues of "power" and "control" in the therapeutic relationship and implicitly speaks to the issue of power and control in client relationships with others and with voices. Your clients can generalize the experience of being able to set limits, give direction, and be empowered in the therapeutic relationship to their relationships outside of therapy and with their voices.

Engagement: Points to Remember

Below we discuss a number of important areas to consider in the therapeutic engagement process. These include building trust, developing agency, control and empowerment, enhancing strengths and skills, honoring the meaning and function of clients' experiences, addressing potential therapeutic barriers, and finally enhancing an empowering understanding of the past and how it relates to the present. As previously discussed, therapeutic engagement and alliance building is not static. It continues throughout the therapy process.

Build Trust

- Safety, trust, compassion, and empathy are paramount. This may be one of the first times clients have been able to share their experience while experiencing another person's understanding and validation. Start with safer material first.

Develop Agency, Control, and Empowerment

- Put your clients in the driver's seat with respect to pace, speed, frequency, venue, and depth of exploration. Enhance self-efficacy and empowerment in your clients by giving them control over appropriate areas of the therapy.

- Never go too fast. The experience of safety in the therapeutic relationship, including understanding and a sense of the valuing of your clients' lived experience, is critical. A client may take multiple sessions, months, or even years to share about certain experiences.

- Respect your clients' right to not share details and aspects that they do not feel comfortable or safe sharing at this time. Here are some comments and questions that can be helpful: "I'm so glad you let me know." "Thank you for letting me know that you don't feel comfortable sharing this right now." "This therapy is for you and we want to go at a pace that feels right for you." "Is there anything getting in the way of you discussing this?" "What would need to be different for you to share more?" "Perhaps we can come back to this later in the therapy."

Enhance Strengths and Skills

- Inform your client that symptoms may get worse at the very start of therapy and at other times during the therapy. Work on grounding and other emotion regulation strategies that can be used both during the therapy session and/or between sessions.

- Take a strengths-focused, normalizing, and value-driven recovery approach that engenders motivation and hope.

- Develop coping and emotion regulation skills as a foundation for assessment and therapeutic work; build on these key skills and integrate them throughout therapy.

- Work on self-valuing and self-compassion (as well as trust) can impact powerfully on the distress, content, and frequency of symptoms. A challenging stance is neither a clinically useful nor advisable approach, as it can create distance between you and your client and contribute to greater "entrenchment" on the part of your client.

Honor the Meaning and Function of Client Experiences

- Honor the current purpose and meaning of your client's experiences and symptoms. For example, voices may serve a compensatory role. Hearing voices can make a client who struggles with low self-esteem feel special. Voices can also serve as company to stave off loneliness. The experience of having a psychotic illness is frequently very isolating and marginalizing. Voices may be experienced as friends or entertainment. In addition, clients may withdraw to avoid symptoms. It is essential to have full, informed consent from your client prior to commencing assessment and therapy. And it is critical to focus on values and valued life goals to address the meaning and purpose the symptoms and voices may serve. Value and goal work with your client can address gaps and potential compensatory functions of symptoms.

- Before working to shift understanding, experience of, and relationship with symptoms and voices, the role that symptoms and voices serve must be addressed.

- Adopt a stance of curiosity about your clients' experience and the meaning of the experiences and symptoms to your clients.

Address Potential Therapeutic Barriers

- Be alert for instances when you, as clinician, are incorporated into beliefs, delusions, and voices. Also be alert for potential commentary by the voices about the therapy or you as clinician.

- Be aware of the possibility that voices may threaten clients who discuss their voices. Address these possibilities in a proactive, transparent, and collaborative manner prior to starting assessment and therapy, thereby developing an agreed upon action plan should these issues occur in therapy.

- Be watchful for signs of the symptoms, such as voices, distracting clients in session, which may impact client concentration and understanding.

Enhance Understanding of the Past and How It Relates to the Present

- Highlight coping strategies or strengths that clients have used at times of difficulty in the past.

- Validate what your clients have been through.

- Emphasize client courage and resiliency—both in the past and currently.

- Reinforce that your clients were doing what they could at the time.

- Normalize by indicating that your clients' responses were understandable given their pervious experiences or the situation at the time.

- Be alert to and highlight client strengths, coping strategies, and circumstances that are different now.

Engagement: What *Not* to Do

Clinicians can sometimes be under time pressures or have misperceptions about how to engage in a therapeutic manner. We find a collaborative pacing and approach in therapy is best. It is important to err on the side of caution by proceeding slowly to ensure safety and trust. Below we highlight some of the key things *not* to do in therapy.

- Provide insufficient time for developing rapport and safety.

- Take a challenging stance or tone.

- Try to convince, lecture, or argue.

- Have a hierarchical educational stance.

- Take a me-you stance.

- Focus on *your* goals or agenda instead of that of your client.

- Focus on symptoms and *not* the whole person and the person's lived experience.

- Ignore the client's strengths, qualities, and successes.

- Try to prove that you are right and your client's understanding is wrong.

- Use language that your client cannot relate to or finds pathologizing.

- Resist individualizing and pacing your therapy work.

- Criticize noncompletion of homework or issues with attendance or punctuality.

- Forget to address safety and appeasement behaviors.

- Overlook trauma history.

- Lose hope.

The what-*not*-to-do list above serves as a reminder of the importance of a collaborative, nonconfrontational, and nonjudgmental approach to engagement and therapy. Implicit in this therapeutic approach is a respectful, strengths-focused, and compassionate relationship and stance with clients.

Initial Assessment

This section covers the main components of the initial meeting. We will consider informed consent, initial history, and assessment.

Informed Consent

The history should be conducted collaboratively within the context of the therapeutic relationships. As with any therapeutic relationship, fully informed consent, including potential benefits and drawbacks, is required. We often discuss how, at times, symptoms may increase in therapy, while proactively addressing how these will be handled. Consent can be presented in the least threatening manner possible by indicating that this is a standard procedure that you, as the clinician, need to go over with clients. You may find it helpful to use statements like "Please humor me," "Please bear with me," "I realize you have probably discussed this before," or "I value our relationship and getting your input and consent is important to me." An agreement as to how, as clinician and client, you would like to address any issues related to risk, reached collaboratively early on in therapy, should be discussed at the outset and emphasize how you value maintaining rapport, safety, and client input. Indicate that, if you are concerned about risk, you will speak to clients first, if possible. However, if this is not possible, due to caring for your clients and your need to keep your clients safe, you will use your professional judgment to get help for your clients. Indicate that this may mean you talking to their physician or the two of you going to the hospital emergency together. At this point, rapport can be enhanced by discussing any ideas clients have around addressing risk and what has been helpful in the past. It can be helpful to ask directly how you can maintain the best rapport possible if these types of approaches are required due to concerns about risks. Again, discussions around risk need to be tailored for each therapeutic relationship. As clinician, you need to be vigilant for the potential for an increase in suspicious thoughts, paranoia, or concerns regarding trust and safety when risk issues are discussed.

Initial History and Assessment

Beck and colleagues (2009) give an excellent suggested outline for the initial history or evaluation (see form 4.1). Areas covered include examination information, general client information and life history—including the individual's own early childhood, family, school, and social history (of which history of trauma is a critical piece), as well as more detailed information about individual and family psychiatric history—and current problems and concerns, health habits, physical health, current personal and social life, current and past treatment, attitude toward treatment, and other observations. Consistent with our strengths-based model, we weave discussion around personal strengths, qualities, skills, coping strategies, and resources throughout the initial interview and throughout therapy. Of course, assessment and conceptualization are an ongoing part of the therapy process. The conceptualization is dynamic and evolving based on new information, client willingness to share, and client changes. History taking and assessment are part of the intervention process and can be experienced as therapeutic if done skillfully.

Information is collected with an eye to beliefs about self, others, the world, and the future; beliefs and attitudes toward symptoms and illness; and strategies, including control and safety behaviors, used to deal with problems. Clients have typically developed helpful and unhelpful strategies for coping with distress and symptoms. The role of experiential avoidance, trying to control thoughts or voices, and safety behaviors such as using a special ritual to deal with voices should be explored. Key elements of the history are trauma, substance use, risk to self and others, and the associated plan to address risk (with special attention to command hallucinations; see chapter 9). The exploration and definition of values and valued life goals is initiated and remains ongoing. Identification of values and valued directions is motivating and enhances hope and engagement. The cognitive behavioral assessment includes cognitive, behavioral, emotional, and physiological processes as well as attention to environmental influences. Prepsychosis beliefs and precipitators at the time of the first experience of psychosis should be explored. In addition, the general constellation of predisposing, precipitating, perpetuating, and protective factors should be addressed—this information is important for relapse prevention and understanding your client's relapse signature. Key cognitive components to address include attention, intrusions, distortions, and imagery. Key behavioral components to cover include avoidance, escape, and safety behaviors. The information gleaned from the history, assessment, and work on values and valued life goals provides much of the initial material for the conceptualization and treatment plan that is described in chapter 5. To facilitate assessment, a list of selected assessment measures can be found on our website (http://www.treatingpsychosis.com) and a list of areas to cover in the assessment can be found in form 4.1. Although assessment is ongoing throughout therapy, important areas to cover in the initial assessment include the problem list (and associated treatment goals) and the strengths, coping strategies, and resources list (see form 4.3). The strengths list should be a living document, as the identification, enhancement, and development of strengths, accomplishments, and resources are an integral part of the treatment model, approach, and goals.

Feedback from Client on the Session

Ask your clients for feedback from the session. Check in regarding current emotions and level of distress given material covered in the session(s). Ask if your clients have any questions or concerns or anything to add. Discuss with your clients how it felt for them to share their story with you. Ask if there was anything you did or said that upset or bothered them. Indicate that you will be asking for such input in each session to try to ensure the therapy is as collaborative, positive, and helpful as possible for your client. Throughout each session, solicit both positive and constructive feedback from your clients as well as clarification for understanding.

Summary of Session

Briefly summarize what was covered in the session and thank your clients for sharing their story. Discuss the importance of the history and storytelling process for the therapeutic process. Highlight client accomplishments, coping strategies, courage, and resilience. Begin to complete form 4.3 collaboratively with your clients to highlight strengths, coping strategies, and resources. In each subsequent session, add additional information to form 4.3. It will serve as a base for the staying well plan developed at the completion of therapy (see chapter 10).

Coping or Grounding Exercise

Provide the rationale for conducting a coping or grounding exercise at the end of the session. See form 4.2 for a selection of coping or grounding exercises. After providing a rationale for completing the grounding exercise at home in between sessions, ask your clients if they would be willing to try the grounding exercise two to three times each day, doing the exercise for two to five minutes each time. (See form 4.2 for client instructions.) If your clients seem hesitant, explore any hesitancy, and reduce the frequency and/or length of the practice based on client input. Indicate that there is no right or wrong, pass or fail; the exercise is about being curious and checking out what can be discovered and/or what may be helpful to them. Indicate that you will try the grounding exercise as well and then check in at the next session to see how it went. It can be helpful for your understanding of the difficulties inherent in following through on between-session practice to try the practice out yourself each week.

Then share your experience of the between-session practice when you review it together in the subsequent therapy session.

Additional Resources

For more information, please see the Resources section of this book. You will find many of the forms in the appendix; they are also available for download at http://www.newharbinger.com/24076. (See the back of this book for instructions on how to access them.) Additional materials not available in this book can be found on our website at http://www.treatingpsychosis.com.

CHAPTER 5

Module 2: Conceptualization and Treatment Planning: Strengths, Values, and Goals

This module can be broken down into therapy sessions based on the individual needs of your client. For group interventions, conceptualization should be done as part of the pregroup assessment—and ongoing as well, of course! Although addressed in the pregroup assessment, values, goals, strengths and resources, and the treatment plan are an integral part of the group material and group process.

Materials

See appendix for forms. They are also available for download at http://www.newharbinger.com/24076. (See the back of this book for instructions on how to access them.)

Modifications for Group Implementation

Ideally, the history and assessment should be completed by the group leader(s) in the individual pre-group orientation and assessment. The pregroup meeting(s) should help group members begin to identify personal values and goals that will then be consolidated in the group. Consistent with the treatment model, a strengths-based approach to assessment is taken. This includes beginning the development of a strengths, coping strategies, and resources list (see form 4.3) as well as development of the list of problems or barriers identified in the conceptualization and development of goals. The group leaders and clients will also begin to develop a conceptualization and treatment plan in the pre-group meeting(s). Values, goals, and conceptualization can be continued as part of the group process. It can be extremely beneficial for group members to write down values and goals on an index card, and for the group leaders to put group members' values and goals on a poster on the group room wall. Conceptualization is an ongoing process within the group as additional themes arise for each group member and core beliefs or schemas are addressed.

Goals and Outline of Module (2 to 4 sessions, and ongoing)

This chapter continues on the history taking and assessment in module 1. It also focuses on creating an individualized case conceptualization; assessing and constructing values; developing short- and long-term goals; identifying your client's strengths, coping strategies, and resources; developing a list of barriers or problems; and collaboratively developing a treatment plan.

Overview of Treatment Area for Clinician

Review the module prior to the session, including any handouts and relevant additional resources in the Resources section and companion website at http://www.treatingpsychosis.com.

Rationale for Development of Values, Goals, Conceptualization, and Treatment Plan

Check-In

At the beginning of each session, complete a check-in with clients based on their functioning since the last session, including the day of the current session. The check-in can involve these four ratings:

Mood rating 0–10 (10 being the highest level of positive mood)

Anxiety rating 0–10 (10 being the highest level of anxiety)

Self-efficacy or accomplishment rating 0–10 (10 being the highest level of self-efficacy)

Psychosis rating 0–10 (10 constituting the highest level of distress associated with thoughts or delusions and/or hallucinations such as voices).

Summary and Link to Previous Session

Ask your clients how they felt during and after the last session. Given that you discussed their past history, distressing affect may have been activated. Address any issues or concerns. Ask if there was anything important that you did not discuss or anything they would like to add. Reinforce strengths and coping strategies that came from the assessment, and ask your clients if they would be willing to continue this session by focusing on values and goals in order to develop a treatment plan together.

Review and Problem-Solving of Between-Session Practice

Ask your clients if they tried completing the grounding exercise(s) at home since the last session. Process how the exercise(s) went. Reinforce what was completed. Normalize and problem-solve any difficulties your clients had. If they did not try the exercise, model a curious stance to discover what got in the way. Use the analogy of exercise or eating a healthier diet, and indicate that just as we wouldn't expect to be a star skier or be in top shape after one day of exercise or skiing, so too grounding, coping, and other strategies in this treatment are skills that we develop over time with practice and that benefits may not show themselves for quite a while—weeks or even months. Tie this in with the focus on values in today's session and the role of personal values in motivating us to engage in what is important to us.

Coping Exercise

As in all sessions, a therapeutic way to begin the session is to lead a short (two- to five-minute) coping or mindfulness exercise. We recommend doing one of the the grounding exercises in the first few sessions (see form 4.2) followed by other coping exercises. It is essential to explore your clients' experience after the exercise. Helpful process questions for mindfulness, coping, and compassion exercises are provided on the companion website at http://www.treatingpsychosis.com.

Overview of Session/Topic Area for Clients

Provide a brief overview of the session content and rationale. Indicate to your clients that you will give them the Session Summary form to take home at the end of the session (see form 5.1). Ask your clients to write down any additions, questions, and barriers to between-session practice on the summary form. Tailor pacing and content to client functioning on the day of the session. Take breaks or finish early as required based on client input. Provide a rationale for covering today's session material for the session exercises.

Clinician Stance

As in the previous session, highlight coping strategies or strengths. Focus on meaning and developing a more fulfilling life. Bring a hopeful stance to the list of barriers or problems that you develop with your clients. Speak to the benefits that others with similar issues have experienced in trying these approaches. Encourage use of the Session Summary (form 5.1) in each session to help consolidate gains and both cue and encourage between-session practice.

Module Therapeutic Strategies and Exercises

In ACT, Hayes, Strosahl, and Wilson (1999) define *values* as "verbally construed global desired life consequences" (p. 206). Within the context of therapy, values are qualities or ways of behaving that the individual engages in to pursue meaningful or valued life goals. Thus, the ultimate goal of therapy in our integrated treatment model is pursuing a value-consistent life, which involves working toward developing a more meaningful life.

Conceptualization

The clinical conceptualization is crucial for the treatment plan and serves as a guide for the treatment process. The conceptualization is like a road map or compass that helps guide the direction of therapy. When uncertain about how to proceed in therapy, revisiting the conceptualization can be extremely helpful for providing direction. The conceptualization should be completed collaboratively with your clients. It should be revised based on new information, insights, or change, as the conceptualization process is dynamic, and shifts throughout therapy due to increased understanding and changes made within therapy.

The initial history is a critical piece of the conceptualization process. Through collaborative and caring exploration of client history, it is possible for you and your clients to develop a shared understanding of how past experiences have impacted them and the development of both healthy and unhealthy core beliefs about self, others (the world), and the future. Frequently, the conceptualization process has focused on unhealthy or maladaptive core beliefs. However, in our positive psychology–infused approach to treatment, we integrate a focus on healthy or adaptive core beliefs to leverage engagement, shift the perspective and experience of our clients, and foster meaningful change. The history, assessment, and conceptualization process can be a therapeutic experience in and of itself as it focuses on strengths, coping strategies, and resources. Conceptualization is usually conducted collaboratively. It initially starts from hypotheses that the clinician develops during history taking, and it evolves over the therapy. Typically, it can be helpful to start with the CBT triangle of thoughts, emotions, and behaviors, using an example generated by your client. Following psychoeducational work on the CBT triangle and the role of physiological or physical sensations, fill in relevant information with your clients from the history, thought records, and clinical exploration clarifying core beliefs and associated rules. *Rules* are typically "if-then" statements. For example, "If I hide my true self, then people will not reject me" or "If I am silent, then people won't punish or hurt me." The conceptualization can be completed collaboratively with your clients as a working document that is referred to, elaborated on, and changed, based on new insights, information, and progress. The conceptualization can be completed together on a whiteboard or piece of paper for your client to take home. (Figure 5.1 shows the conceptualization form. See figure 5.2 for a sample completed conceptualization; see form 5.2 for a blank conceptualization form that can be used with your clients.) Timing, pacing, and the collaborative style used to develop the conceptualization varies by individual and is based on clinical judgment. Whenever you or your clients feel lost in therapy, it can be extremely helpful to revisit the conceptualization so as to assess your progress and your approach to therapeutic goals.

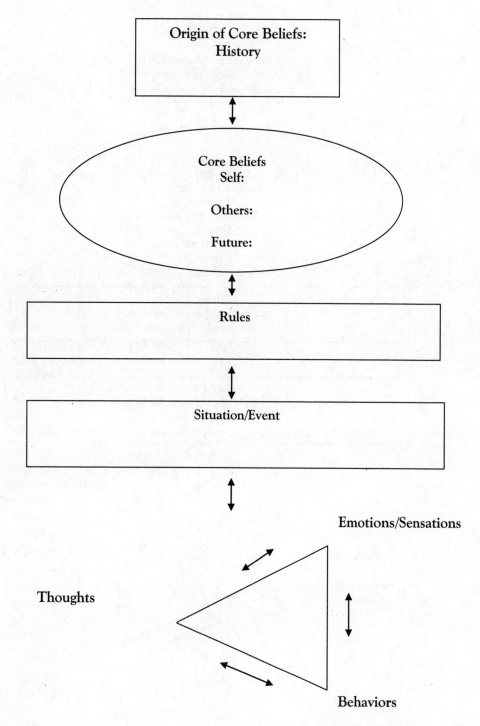

FIGURE 5.1   Cognitive Behavioral Conceptualization. (Modified with permission from Beck, 1995.)

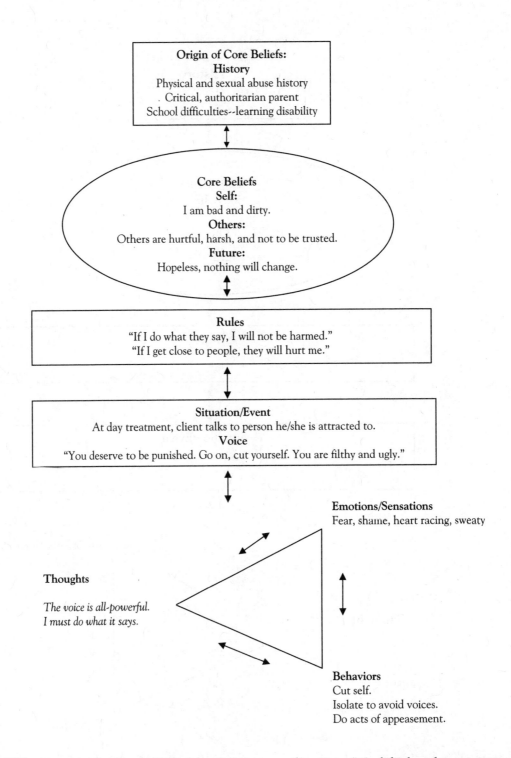

FIGURE 5.2   Sample Cognitive Behavioral Conceptualization. (Modified with permission from Beck, 1995.)

The conceptualization process includes not only challenges and areas for growth but also a parallel focus on strengths, qualities, coping strategies, resources, and adaptive core beliefs. A handout on core beliefs (see form 5.3) can be provided and discussed as part of the psychoeducation, conceptualization, and treatment planning process. The conceptualization process also helps in the process of identifying values and goals. The treatment plan develops from the history, assessment, and conceptualization process. However, typically the treatment plan is developed and revisited regularly throughout therapy just as the conceptualization is intricately linked into the therapeutic process.

Values

As Harris (2007) indicates, values are our heart's profound wants and desires. Values can include these elements:

- what we want our life to be about

- what we want to stand for

- what kind of person we want to be

- how we want to behave

- what types of relationships we want to develop

- how we want to relate with others and the world

Values can serve as powerful guides and motivators for client actions—as well as our own, of course! Values are guiding principles that can serve as a map, compass, and motivator for our daily lives. Through identifying and constructing their values, our clients can choose to live in a value-consistent manner and move in valued-life directions.

Values are powerfully connected to life goals but differ from goals per se. Values are the foundation for the valued directions we wish to move in throughout our life. They are a process, and as such are never completed. This is part of the beauty and motivational quality of values because it means they can be accessible at any given moment on any given day through thick and thin, through "good" times and tough times.

After providing an overview about values to your clients, work together in session to complete the Values Worksheet (form 5.4). Read through the definition of values and examples of values on the form. Ask your clients to circle each of the values listed that apply to them. The exercise of endorsing values can be a strengths-oriented and empowering experience in and of itself. Discuss the values that were chosen and ask your clients to narrow the values they have chosen to those that are very important or important to them. Selecting the values that are very important to your clients will help to focus values work without negating the relevance of the other values that were endorsed by your clients. To enhance breadth, discuss values that come from a number of life areas as listed on form 5.4 (leisure, personal development/self-care, education/work (volunteer or paid), and relationships). See http://www.thehappinesstrap.com/free -resources for more examples of values exercises, including bull's-eye worksheets to address degree of value-consistency. In addition, see http://www.acceptandchange.com/materials or http://www.actforado lescents.com/for-professionals/resources-and-freebies for free values cards.

Clinical Tips

It is imperative to address difficulties and barriers to values work. When doing values identification work, it is critical to address issues such as those listed below that can get in the way of meaningful value-based therapeutic work and movement toward valued goals.

- Make sure to clearly differentiate between values and goals. Sometimes these can be confused. For example "I value getting a well-paid job" is a goal, as it does not describe how your client wants to behave.

- Ordering of values work in therapy should be individualized for your clients. You may need to do therapeutic work with beliefs about work with the accuracy or helpfulness of thoughts (defusion) and acceptance before moving on to work with values.

- Explore whether it is your client's own value or a prescribed or societal value. (Often your client will use words such as "should" or "must" associated with prescribed values.)

Clinical Barriers

Values and feelings can be confused. Part of the human experience is that emotional barriers can arise when we are on the path of valued directions and committed action. As Hayes, Strosahl, and Wilson (2012) indicate, remaining consistent with our values even when we may not feel like it at times is important. We provide the clinical example below to highlight the therapeutic processes we have integrated from ACT, CFT, and CBT, including mindfulness and the importance of values in enhancing motivation and reducing emotional and other forms of avoidance.

Clinical Example

Bella, a thirty-four-year-old single woman, has been having fearful and paranoid thoughts and hearing denigrating voices over the past five years. Bella's family emigrated from North Africa to Canada when Bella was a teenager. The family decided to move to Canada after experiencing years of conflict in their country of origin.

Bella spends most of her time in the family home. She goes to appointments with her doctor but otherwise tends not to leave the house. Bella indicates that she stays at home to try to minimize her voices and to avoid the people who she believes are laughing at her and who think she should go back to her country where she belongs. Bella's mother brings her to her first and subsequent therapy appointments.

After a number of therapy sessions, Bella begins to feel more trusting in the relationship with her clinician. When she and her clinician start to discuss what Bella would like her life to be like, Bella talks about her desires to have a boyfriend and to have a job. When values exploration and construction work is done in therapy, it becomes clear that Bella values being a kind and compassionate person in relationships, and that she would like to contribute to her family and to the community by getting a job. When explored further, it becomes clear that Bella's fears of others and her attempt to avoid her voices keep her from important pursuits in her life. (Her behaviors of withdrawing and not going out stop her from disproving her paranoid beliefs and from reinforcing her personal strengths and qualities.)

The values of kindness and compassion in relationship as well as contributing for the benefit of others are identified and highlighted in therapy. Bella's values are (1) to be kind and compassionate in relationships and (2) to make a difference by contributing to her family and community.

When Bella and her clinician consider her values, they also look at her valued goals and the committed actions that she will take to work toward her goals. For example, for Bella's value of making a difference by contributing to her family and community, she selects two goals—one short term and one longer term:

- Go to a fund-raising group at the community center once a week (short term).

- Get a volunteer job at the community center (longer term).

For committed action, Bella makes these choices:

- Do loving-kindness meditation/mindfulness exercises.

- Make self-compassionate coping cards.

- Develop a compassion-for-others coping card.

- Create an image of a caring, kind nurturer.

It becomes clear through therapy that for Bella to be kind and compassionate in her relationships with others, she needs to be kind and compassionate to herself as well. She also needs to allow herself to experience the caring and kindness of others.

Being compassionate is a value that Bella has identified that is important for her to live by and move toward as one of her valued directions. Therefore, her value motivates her to engage in committed action each day to develop and experience compassion for self and others. Bella is then able to start looking at trying to accept that she, like other people, experiences fear and suspiciousness, but she is willing to work on gradually tolerating some of the fear so that she can live a more value-consistent, and ultimately a more meaningful and rich, life.

Bella and Our Integrated Treatment Approach

Let's take a closer look at Bella's experience in therapy. It is an example of the colorful and rich tapestry of our integrated treatment approach in which the treatment, goals, recovery plan, and therapeutic processes are individualized and intertwined.

Bella has a number of sessions with her clinician; she feels heard, validated, and understood. Bella begins to feel more safety and trust within the therapy relationship. Her clinician, through her warmth and strengths-based approach, has helped Bella connect with personal qualities, assets, and coping strategies that she had almost forgotten she had—essentially, the practice of positive psychology. Bella and her clinician collaboratively develop a treatment plan. Bella starts to feel hope in a way she has not in a very long time.

The tapestry of therapy is an unfolding process. Bella identifies that she wants to be compassionate in relationships (a value in ACT). She plans to gradually start doing compassionate actions (B = behaviors in CBT; a compassion-focused behavior in CFT) toward others. This is one of many committed actions that Bella plans to engage in to live more consistently with her identified values. Engaging in committed actions may involve Bella enhancing her acceptance that she will likely continue to have some symptoms or fears but that they will probably get easier to deal with over time. Bella is willing to engage in activities that are compassionate toward herself and others (compassionate behaviors toward self and others in CFT), even if she continues to feel fear. By being willing to try mindfulness exercises (contact with the present moment), Bella can experience herself as an observer of her thoughts, feelings, and sensations. In addition, by considering other explanations and viewpoints (C = cognitions and cognitive reappraisal in CBT; diffusion in ACT) Bella is able to distance from some of her fearful thoughts. By engaging in cognitive reappraisal, Bella can be less fused (enhanced cognitive flexibility through diffusion and/or cognitive reappraisal) with her fearful thoughts that others laugh at her and want her to move away. As a result of living more consistently with her values of being compassionate, Bella starts to feel better about herself and feels less fear about others (emotion in CBT).

With the goal of living a more value-consistent and meaningful life, Bella starts to go out more (behavioral activation, committed action). She increasingly engages in coping strategies and activities that reduce her fear. Bella and her therapist then work on her value of contributing to family and community by planning out the steps needed to help her look for and find a volunteer position and eventually a part-time job. It is Bella's values that have motivated her all along the treatment and recovery path to engage in the self-care, coping strategies, and actions that have enhanced her quality of life.

Goals

A *goal*, unlike a value that serves as a compass or direction, is a desired outcome. It is something one wishes to achieve that has an end point, a finish. Being caring, compassionate, and understanding in one's intimate relationships is a value. Having a girl- or boyfriend, spouse, or partner is a goal. As a goal, marriage can be achieved or completed. But we can achieve a goal and still not live consistently with our values—that is, we can be married and still not be caring, compassionate, and understanding in our relationship. By identifying values, we then proceed to identify valued goals (or vice versa) and committed action required to work toward these goals.

Complete form 5.5 with your clients to establish and clarify goals. Often, cuing clients with what their interests and goals were before their experience of psychosis can be helpful. Collaboratively brainstorm committed action (steps required) to reach both shorter- and longer-term goals. (In chapter 7, we further discuss the activity ladder, or the series of activities to perform in order to achieve goals.)

Consistent with ACT, symptoms can serve as barriers to achieving valued goals and can be addressed in this context—that is, clients may need to experience the affect associated with thoughts, delusions, or voices in order to achieve goals rather than overcoming symptoms as a goal in and of itself. Acceptance of symptoms and distressing emotions can be intricately intertwined in this process rather than the struggle or avoidance that has frequently been associated with delusions and hallucinations. The goal setting form (5.5) is used to set both short- and longer-term goals by identifying SMART goals (specific, measurable, achievable, realistic, and time-limited). Form 5.5 is also used collaboratively to focus on the identification of steps or committed actions required to achieve goals (including barriers to these actions and ways of addressing these barriers or challenges).

Treatment Plan

You and your client collaboratively devise the treatment plan. Although the barriers/problem list serves as a target for areas in which to intervene, an emphasis on strengths, qualities, coping skills, and resources should be an integral part of the treatment planning process. Therefore, the treatment plan includes the strengths, skills, and resources; values; valued short- and long-term goals; the list of problems or potential strategies or interventions to facilitate movement in the direction of valued goals; and the list of barriers or problems. See form 5.6 for the treatment plan. Complete this form collaboratively with your clients based on the values and valued goals you have identified together in forms 5.4 and 5.5, as well as the committed actions required to facilitate achievement of valued goals.

Between-Session Practice

Collaboratively discuss and decide on the between-session practice, clarify understanding, and problem-solve any potential barriers to practice. Using the 0–10 scale (with 0 being least likely and 10 being most likely), ask your clients how likely it is that they will do the between-session practice. Explore and problem-solve reasons for predicted noncompletion and ask your clients to re-rate likelihood of completion, again using the 0–10 scale. Discuss the pros and cons of a reminder phone call or of using cuing devices such as alarms, cell phones, and so on. Give your clients the forms that you have completed together in session, as well as corresponding blank forms on client strengths, values, and goal setting to fill out between session (forms 4.3, 5.4, and 5.5, respectively). Here are two options for between-session practice:

1. Add to the client strengths, coping strategies, and resources list (form 4.3).

2. Complete a coping or grounding exercise between sessions. (Decide collaboratively how long the exercise will be and how many times it should be done before the next session.) Err on the side of providing less practice to enhance the possibility of a successful experience.

Feedback from Client on the Session

Ask your client for constructive feedback on the session. These questions can help to solicit both positive and constructive input from your client at the end of each session as well as enhance transparency and the therapeutic alliance and problem-solve any barriers to therapeutic alliance, engagement, or treatment:

- What was most helpful today/in this session?

- What was least helpful?

- Was there anything you didn't understand or get?

- Was there anything I did or said that bothered you?

- If nothing bothered you, would you be able to let me know if something did bother you? If not, why not?

- Was there anything that didn't fit for you in today's session?

- Was there anything you would like clarification on?

- Was there anything important we forgot to discuss?

- Is there anything you would like to focus on more?

- Is there anything you would like to focus on less?

- On a scale of 0–10, what would you rate this session?

- On a scale of 0–100%, how likely do you think it is that you will come to the next session (0–100%)?

- Do you have any hesitations about this therapy?

- How does this compare to other therapies you have done?

- What would make this therapy better for you?

- What would make this therapy more helpful for you?

- Do you feel upset or worried about anything we discussed?

- Did you notice a change in your voices? If so, how can we handle that?

- What is one thing you will take away from this session?

- What did you like most about this session?

- What did you like least about this session?

- How was the length of the session for you?

- How was the amount of information we covered for you?

- What could I do differently?

- What were the main things you learned in this session?

- How are you feeling right now?

- Would you like to do a grounding or coping exercise?

Summary of Session

Ask your clients to read over the session summary (form 5.1) at home and share this form with family, friends, or caregivers, if they want to. Model a strengths-focused approach by asking your clients to identify one personal strength, quality, or accomplishment from the session, including something they noticed about themselves or tried in the session. If your clients find it difficult to do so, you can cue with examples or ask your clients to think of what a friend or family member might say. Provide your clients with reinforcing, strengths-focused feedback from the session. By focusing on stregnths, qualities, and accomplishments at the beginning and end of each session (as well as throughout), we enhance skills in attending to strengths, acknowledging strengths and accomplishments, and experiencing personal qualities.

Coping Exercise (Optional)

See form 4.2 in the appendix for a selection of coping exercises.

Additional Resources

For more information, please see the Resources section of this book. You will find many of the forms in the appendix; they are also available for download at http://www.newharbinger.com/24076. (See the back of this book for instructions on how to access them.) Additional materials not available in this book can be found on our website at http://www.treatingpsychosis.com.

CHAPTER 6

Module 3: Emotion Regulation and Resilience

This chapter focuses on an integrated treatment approach for emotion regulation and emotional resilience. The chapter flows from the therapeutic work on the identification of strengths, values, valued goals, and committed action discussed in the previous chapter. This module can be broken down into therapy sessions based on the individual needs of your client. It can be implemented as a stand-alone treatment for both individual and group psychotherapy.

Materials

See appendix for forms. They are also available for download at http://www.newharbinger.com/24076. (See the back of this book for instructions on how to access them.) Because the cognitive abilities and needs of clients vary, we've provided additional versions of some forms in this chapter on the New Harbinger website.

Modifications for Group Interventions

The content and strategies in this module are well suited for group interventions. Group discussion of a range of emotions can enhance normalization. In addition, group members can learn from one another regarding strategies to cope with emotions and the ubiquity of distressing experiences and emotions. The use of the term "we" instead of "you" by group leaders at check-in and throughout the group is depathologizing and normalizing of emotions and other experiences. To enhance labeling of emotions, the check-in for each session can involve doing a rating (0–10) for each emotion on the Emotion List (form 6.2). Group processing of exercises can be very powerful for group members to experience universality and being heard, understood, and supported by others.

Goals and Outline of Module (4 to 12 sessions, or longer as clinically appropriate)

In this module, the goal is development and enhancement of foundational coping and emotion regulation skills. The development of these skills is introduced in this module and will be reinforced and enhanced throughout the treatment. This skill development work is needed as a foundation for therapy, for the purposes of stabilization, and to enhance emotional resilience and quality of life. The development and enhancement of emotion regulation skills is also essential prior to proceeding with the middle and later stages of therapy.

Consistent with a trauma-informed approach to treatment, you should have completed a comprehensive assessment that addresses any previous or current experience of trauma (sexual, physical, verbal, or psychological abuse, including bullying). For those with a history of trauma, emotion regulation will likely need to have a greater focus and emphasis. Many clients will have developed emotion regulation strategies to cope with overwhelming affect, overstimulation, and distress. Strategies such as substance use, smoking, cutting, disassociation, gambling, and others may be used, due to a dearth of more adaptive emotion regulation and coping strategies. The strategies listed below can serve as adaptive replacements for emotion regulation strategies such as substance use. A harm reduction approach to substance use, where enhancement of emotion regulation skills is accompanied by a decline in substance use due to the development of alternative, more adaptive coping strategies, can be beneficial. We address the following emotion regulation material and skills in this module:

- Psychoeducation, strengths, and coping skills enhancement

- Normalization and validation

- Acceptance and willingness

- Mindfulness (including flexible present-moment attention or awareness and self-as-observer)

- Compassion-focused therapy approaches

- Cognitive flexibility: cognitive defusion and cognitive reappraisal

- Positive emotions

- Resilience

- Committed action to valued life goals, including a focus on physical and other health strategies (exercise, diet, sleep, smoking, and substance use)

Overview of Treatment Area for Clinician

This section, including any forms and relevant additional resources, should be reviewed by you, as clinician, prior to the session. The emotion regulation strategies covered in this module are in no way exhaustive. For additional emotion regulation strategies, please see "Emotion Regulation and Skills Training" in the Resources section and the companion website http://www.treatingpsychosis.com.

What Is Emotion Regulation?

Emotion regulation refers to the ability to moderate or cope with emotions. Emotion regulation can include a range of coping strategies including confrontation, responsibility taking, distancing, avoiding, self-control, social support, reappraisal, and problem solving (Barlow et al., 2011; Folkman & Lazarus, 1988). Coping strategies for dealing with emotions can either be helpful (adaptive) or unhelpful (maladaptive). In therapy, we aim to foster helpful rather than unhelpful emotion regulation and coping strategies. For example, clients may engage in substance use or yell at voices in an attempt to deal with upsetting emotions. However, these strategies may not be the most life-enhancing and effective ways to cope with distressing emotions. With your clients, collaboratively attempt to identify, develop, and enhance helpful coping strategies to address emotional distress and to modify or replace unhelpful emotion regulation strategies. We refer to emotion regulation and resilience throughout the treatment.

What Is Resilience?

Resilience is defined as successful adaptation to adversity (Zautra, Hall, & Murray, 2010). We have included the term "resilience" to highlight the research literature regarding the helpful and life-enhancing ways one can understand and address adversity, problems, challenges, and difficult emotions. Through strategies that enhance resilience, we can help to empower our clients to enhance and sustain a meaningful life and wellness.

Clinical Considerations: Importance of Values and Valued Goals

In the previous chapter, we discussed the role of values and working toward valued goals in enhancing motivation to engage in helpful and adaptive coping strategies. The therapeutic relationship plays a critical role throughout treatment, as it serves a powerful emotion regulation function. It is important that you empathetically link values and valued goals to the emotion regulation and other therapeutic work. Linking values enhances motivation and engagement in the often-difficult work of awareness of distressing emotions, acceptance of distressing emotions as part of being human, and implementation of helpful emotion regulation strategies. Although we may prefer not to have upsetting emotions, the engendering of emotion regulation strategies can replace experiential avoidance. As a therapist, you engage in a delicate dance with your client by encouraging exposure to distressing emotions or experiences, including thoughts, feelings, and physical sensations, while respecting your client's personal agency, effectiveness, and pacing. By individualized collaborative pacing, the "work" of therapy can be conducted within the "therapeutic window," which is ideally experienced by your client as neither too overwhelming nor too overstimulating or activating. As therapist, you model a compassionate, curious, and empowering stance. Our therapeutic approach is informed by positive psychology and a recovery approach that emphasizes client strengths, self-identified values, and valued goals. As in ACT, it is critical to consistently work with personal values to engage your clients in the variety of therapeutic approaches used throughout treatment: behavioral activation; traditional CBT for psychosis; and compassion-focused, mindfulness-based, and acceptance and commitment-based strategies. The focus of such work with values is not on emotion control but on understanding, experiencing, and accepting emotions as they are. Through consistent work with personal vaules, and strategies to enhance efficacy in coping with distressing emotions, your clients become better able to direct energy to pursuing valued directions and goals.

Rationale for Development of Emotion Regulation Skills

The first stage of therapy—the development of emotion regulation skills and resilience—is essential. This work is foundational, but, by necessity, it is also woven through the therapy. Emotion regulation skills serve not only as a platform, or base, to work from but also as skills to be enhanced, reinforced, and reintroduced to deal with distressing affect that arises as a function of everyday stressors, the treatment process, and the often nonlinear course of experiencing psychoses.

Emotion regulation work is required to address the experiencing, processing, and expressing of emotions. As Khoury and Lecomte (2012) indicate, individuals who have a diagnosis of schizophrenia experience higher levels of subjective distress in response to stressors. In addition, research indicates that individuals who experience psychosis tend to use less helpful methods of dealing with stressful emotions, such as avoidance, suppression, rumination, and worry (Khoury & Lecomte, 2012). Given that those with a diagnosis of schizophrenia have greater difficulties with perception and recognition of emotions as well as interpretation of emotion within a social context (including recognition of verbal and facial emotional cues), development of social and emotional skills is an important focus. Research (see Khoury & Lecomte, 2012) indicates that individuals with psychosis tend to have greater difficulty in understanding the intentions and emotional state of others (in what's known as theory of mind). These challenges with experiencing, understanding, and expressing emotions speak to the need to address these areas of difficulty in therapy. In addition, given the difficulties with both facial and verbal expression of emotion, others may not realize the emotional experience of those with psychosis and may not respond accordingly.

Individuals with psychosis predict less pleasure and mastery with respect to social situations (Beck et al., 2009). These so-called "defeatist" beliefs can contribute to social isolation, decreased engagement, and limited practice of social skills. As a result, individuals receive less corrective feedback, thereby reinforcing defeatist beliefs (Beck et al., 2009).

Therefore, it is important to address these emotional and social difficulties. It is critical to enhance skills in dealing with the emotions or distress that precede and exacerbate symptoms and/or setbacks and that will be experienced as a part of therapy and day-to-day life in working toward valued goals. It is important to educate clients that, consistent with an approach that involves working toward valued goals, emotions and/or symptoms may increase at times ("no pain, no gain"). That is, distress, often manifested in the form of symptoms, will increase at times during the course of therapy, in the service of working toward valued goals.

Emotion regulation skills will be required within the session, in day-to-day life, and, of course, during application of different types of "real-life practice" or homework, including working with experiential avoidance and exposure. In addition, development of these grounding and affect regulation skills enables your clients to experience efficacy and agency. These skills allow your clients to have the experience of being able to accept and stay with distressing experiences and symptoms and cope with the associated affect. Consistent with an approach that is not overwhelming or overstimulating, the work both in sessions and out is maintained within a "therapeutic window" that does not overwhelm your client emotionally and physiologically (Courtois & Ford, 2012). An approach to therapy that involves working within a "therapeutic window" of exposure to emotion enables your clients to, if necessary, slow the pace of the session and to discontinue the discussion or exercises. Given that clients who have psychoses have higher rates of trauma than average and can feel overstimulated and overwhelmed by emotions, working within this therapeutic window is essential. By working within the therapeutic window, affect and the corresponding physiological activation and sensations are maintained within a manageable range. By preparing your clients for an increase in distressing affect during the course of treatment, increases in emotion are normalized, expected, planned for, and problem-solved proactively, thereby decreasing the likelihood of dropout.

Research Alert

Research (see Khoury & Lecomte, 2012) indicates that although clients may look like they have "flat affect" or are not experiencing emotion, they experience an equivalent amount of emotion to others; but it frequently is neither verbalized nor shown through facial and other nonverbal expression. In fact, a higher level of subjective distress is reported in response to stressors. Importantly, it has been found that those with psychosis experience equivalent positive emotion, but they do not anticipate this and are not able to maintain this positive emotion for as long as others.

Agenda for the Session

Discuss the agenda for the session with your clients. Collaboratively decide on the amount of content and number of skills to be covered in the session, including time for check-in and for addressing any issues that may have arisen, including any issues of a more urgent nature, as well as review and problem solving of between-session practice. Any issues that have come up can be placed on the agenda and linked to the session topic and content. Pacing is essential. Checking in with your clients for feedback both during and at the end of the session facilitates appropriate pacing of the sessions and material covered. Pacing and individualization often address overstimulation; however, checking in for feedback can also provide the opportunity for clients to give input when pacing is too slow or not engaging. To facilitate collaboration, ask your clients in each session whether there is anything they would like to put on the agenda.

Check-In

Complete a check-in with your clients based on their functioning since the last session, including the day of the current session. The check-in can involve the following ratings:

Mood rating 0–10 (10 being the highest level of positive mood)

Anxiety rating 0–10 (10 being the highest level of anxiety)

Self-efficacy or accomplishment rating 0–10 (10 being the highest level of self-efficacy or accomplishment)

Psychosis rating 0–10 (10 constituting the highest level of distress associated with thoughts, delusions, and/or hallucinations, such as voices). A power rating can also be conducted to gage the power differential with voices (0–10, with 10 being the highest level of power attributed to voices).

Summary and Link to Previous Session

Ask your clients what they recall from the last session. Reinforce what was recalled, and normalize **any** difficulties with remembering material from session to session. Summarize the material from the previous session and link it to the between-session practice and this session's topic.

Review and Problem Solving of Between-Session Practice

Ask your clients about their experience with doing the between-session practice. Reinforce what was completed. Empathetically normalize any difficulties your clients had with the practice. Collaboratively problem-solve any of the barriers or difficulties raised.

Coping Exercise

Lead your clients in one of the coping and/or grounding exercises (form 4.2). Be aware of any potential issues for clients with a history of trauma around bodywork (e.g., the body scan). Provide an opportunity for clients to experience a diversity of coping exercises by doing different exercises in each session. Alternatively, you can collaboratively decide with your clients if they would prefer to repeat the same coping exercise a number of times or throughout the therapy. Exercises highlighting the transitory nature of emotions can be beneficial at this point. For example, the coping exercise on thoughts and feelings as waves on the ocean or clouds passing in the sky can be illustrative at this point in therapy. Urge and emotion surfing are constructs that can also be helpful to clients now.

Overview of Session/Topic Area for Clients

Provide a brief overview of the session content and rationale. The content should be targeted at the appropriate level for your clients and the amount of content tailored for your clients. Individualization is key!

Clinician Stance

Your stance should be one of understanding, compassion, and encouragement. It is also important to be open and curious about the exploration of emotions.

Module Therapeutic Strategies and Exercises

This module contains nine content areas. These can be completed in nine sessions, or in whichever number of sessions is therapeutically appropriate for your clients. The therapeutic strategies discussed in this module are integrated from CBT, CFT, ACT, and mindfulness orientations or approaches. At first glance, clinicians may question the integration of approaches from different theoretical backgrounds; however, we have found the integration of these approaches to have a synergistic effect. In the material that follows, we see values work as an intrinsic motivator in working toward valued goals and living a richer, more meaningful life. Although the goal is not change for change's sake (or the removal of "symptoms"), change frequently occurs as a result of engaging in many of the processes or approaches below as clients move in the direction of valued goals. We incorporate strategies that are "helpful" or "workable" in living a more value-consistent and meaningful life. Symptoms may temporarily increase as a result of decreasing emotional or experiential avoidance and heightened contact with distressing emotions. When we discuss acceptance, we recognize both "positive" and "negative" emotions and focus on the workability of enhancing the experience of positive emotions and personal strengths while at the same time not engaging in avoidance around "negative" emotions or qualities.

Psychoeducation, Strengths, and Coping Skills Enhancement

This section focuses on understanding emotions. We focus on emotions in the context of the thought-emotion-behavior triad as described in chapter 5 (module 2). Helping your clients make the connection among thoughts, feelings, and behavior enhances their understanding of emotions as well as their sense of efficacy and agency in coping with emotions. By understanding the links among thoughts, feelings, physical sensations, and behaviors (including emotion-driven behaviors), your clients can learn to influence their emotional experiences. Given that those who experience psychosis often have difficulties or deficits in the experiencing, processing, and expressing of emotion, enhancing client understanding of emotions through psychoeducation and experiential exercises is extremely important.

—FORM 6.1: Understanding Emotions

Discuss the handout on understanding emotions collaboratively with your clients. Ask for an example of a situation in which a strong emotion came up. Through their personal example, help your clients to make connections among their thoughts, behaviors, and emotions. It is important to use an example from client experience. If your clients are not able to come up with an example, cue them based on a distressing situation or emotion you have discussed in the past. This way any questions and misconceptions can be addressed in session, and you can determine client understanding of the information discussed regarding emotions. At times, clients may have difficulty recognizing that an emotion is their own. For example, clients unaccustomed to experiencing emotion in general, or a particular type of emotion, due to anhedonia or blunted affect may misattribute an emotion to an external cause, such as a voice.

—FORM 6.2: Emotion List

Review the Emotion List in session with your clients. Discuss each of the emotions on the list and ask your clients if they experience this emotion. Discuss the importance of noticing and labeling emotions to gain a better understanding of emotions and how to deal with them. Noticing and recording emotions is important to enhance emotion granulation skills in psychosis. Clients with psychosis may have greater difficulty distinguishing between or labeling different emotions (what's known as *granulation of emotions*). They may say something like "I feel bad" but not label the specific emotion any further. If your clients have any difficulties, give examples from your previous discussions, your own experience, or more generic examples. For instance, you might say, "What emotion would you feel if you saw a person (or animal) that was hurt?" "What emotion do you think a friend might feel if he or she saw a person (or animal) that was hurt?"

Coping Strategies

Consistent with the strengths focus in therapy, initiate discussion by asking your clients about the strategies they currently use to deal with distressing emotions and tie these in with their strengths, values, and goals. For example, if your client says, "I remind myself that this feeling will pass," you might say, "Great, so it sounds like you use self-coaching. How does that work for you?" Your client may then respond by saying, "It helps some of the time." You might respond by saying, "Fabulous, so you already have a coping strategy that works for you. Now we can work together to find other coping strategies that might help you." By identifying existing strategies, therapy can focus on enhancing the use of "helpful" emotion regulation strategies and starting to explore the potential costs and benefits of strategies that are not so helpful (for example, avoidance, suppression, using substances, and so on). See form 6.3, Strategies for Coping with Emotions. Please note: encourage your clients to add coping strategies that they find helpful from form 6.3 to their strengths, coping strategies, and resources list (form 4.3).

If your clients have difficulty coming up with coping strategies, you can cue them with a list of strategies commonly used to cope with emotions (see form 6.3). It is important that the discussion of emotions addresses both "positive" or "pleasant" and "negative" or "unpleasant" emotions, and that it highlights the role of a full range of emotional experiences and the adaptive function that "negative" emotions can often play (for example, anger may mean that a right has been violated; fear can help energize the client in a dangerous situation). Given that clients who experience psychosis often have difficulties identifying emotions, cuing and discussion of facial expressions can be helpful.

Any difficulties your clients have in differentiating between thoughts and feelings can be addressed by informing your clients that emotions are often one word. Giving the following statement to fill in can help: "I felt _____ [joy, fear, sad, happy]." If any difficulties occur, a normalizing statement can be helpful: for example, "Lots of people find it difficult to identify emotions and know the difference between thoughts and feelings. I had a hard time figuring it out at first [only if this is true for you]. We can figure it out together. It does get easier."

Clinical Consideration: Increase in Symptoms

As in any type of therapy, symptoms such as voices may actually increase initially and/or at different times during the therapy process. Therefore, it is important to indicate to your clients that symptoms (and distressing affect) can increase at times in therapy.

You and your clients can then problem-solve how an increase in symptoms or distressing affect can be dealt with, thereby reducing premature termination or concerns regarding the benefits of therapy. In addition, the work on the enhancement and development of coping skills and affect regulation strategies in this module can be emphasized, practiced, and reinforced by you from session to session. The use of strategies, such as a hand signal indicating stop or a "panic button," is both respectful and empowering. Through these types of strategies, your clients have control over the pace at which therapy is conducted, the ability to take a break or disengage at any time, and the agency to reengage when ready. Discuss *beforehand* what entails a workable increase in distress and the importance of continuing—for example, in an exposure exercise, premature cessation might amplify fear over the long run and increase beliefs regarding an inability to cope with fear. Using a previously agreed upon graded approach that is paced based on client input is essential.

Clinical Consideration: Trust, Safety, and Pacing

As always, trust, safety, and pacing are critical in a compassionate, trauma-informed approach to care. Given the elevated history of abuse in those with psychosis, you should scan for any verbal or nonverbal signs of distress or triggering, such as emotional dysregulation or overstimulation and activation. You should also monitor for disconnection in session, apparent preoccupation with voices, and nonverbal signs of distress or withdrawal—for example, reduced eye contact, increased paucity of speech, repetitive movements or gestures, and so on. At this point, gentle inquiry to identify distress and develop coping strategies is important. Examples of helpful questions include these: "What's going on for you right now?" "How is this pacing for you?" "Please let me know if I touch on anything that is very upsetting to you." "Can you write down or draw what you are feeling (or what is going on for you), if you can't put it in words?" "Would you like to take a break?" Starting and ending each session with identification of a personal strength and a grounding exercise helps to contain affect and increase a sense of self-efficacy.

Normalization and Validation

Normalization and validation are part of the psychoeducation process and the therapy as a whole. Normalizing and depathologizing are important components of an empathetic and engaging approach to working with emotions. Given that those who experience psychosis have often had their experiences invalidated or discounted, the clinician's understanding, empathetic support, and nonjudgmental curiosity are key. For clients sharing unusual thoughts, delusions, and experiences (hearing voices, seeing things, and so on) that are not experiences shared by others (for example, "spies are watching me"), try to get an understanding of what that must be like for them. Statements such as "That must be very difficult for you" can validate the person's experience without having a "colluding" quality. You can then notice emotional themes and normalize and validate these themes.

Kingdon and Turkington (1991) first described the crucial importance of a normalizing explanation for psychotic symptoms in CBT for schizophrenia. Psychotic symptoms such as hallucinations and delusions are conceptualized as falling on the end of a continuum with "normal" experience. Hallucinations and delusions are viewed as within the range of normal experience but involve a catastrophic or inaccurate appraisal of physiological sensations, self-talk, and cognitive intrusions.

—FORM 6.1: Understanding Emotions

Revisit and review form 6.1 on understanding emotions, physical sensations, thoughts, and psychotic experiences. Discuss any misunderstandings or misperceptions regarding the material and validate the emotion that often accompanies these experiences. Emotions can be modeled by the therapist for identification and discussion; or, pre-prepared DVD clips illustrating emotional states can be shown. The clips are particularly useful as they can be chosen to illustrate emotional acceptance and expression in strategic ways, beginning with less challenging emotions such as sadness and leading up to anxiety, anger, and shame. Clients might want to practice the scenes depicted as a means of exploring affective expression in a decentered format. Role reversal and even group enactment of scenes from the clips might follow.

—COPING CARDS

Collaboratively generate more normalizing ways of understanding emotions and the client's psychotic experiences. These alternative explanations can then be written on coping cards. *Coping cards* record self-generated coping statements. (See our website http://www.treatingpsychosis.com for examples.) The statements are typically written on index cards, which can be carried in a pocket or purse, to make them easily accessible when clients are distressed or feeling overwhelmed. Coping cards can include positive affirmations ("I'm a good person; I don't need to believe what the voices say"), normalizing statements ("Lots of people hear voices"), coping statements ("I can handle my voices"), and skills or coaching statements ("Remember to use your compassionate imagery"). Coping cards can be written in the client's own words and handwriting or in the clinician's words and handwriting, whichever is preferred. Coping cards are deceptively simple, but we have found them to be an incredibly powerful therapeutic tool. Audio and video recordings can also be used to reinforce coping.

Clinical Consideration: Curious and Nondiscounting Stance

Validation and normalization are helpful engagement and empathy-enhancing processes. For clients, the thoughts and experiences are real—that is, clients who report hearing voices have an experience that they label as a voice. The voice-hearing experience is not shared by others, but it is nonetheless an experience that clients have that has thoughts and emotions associated with it. A curious and nondiscounting stance on your part is important. You may be asked by your clients whether you believe their experience (for example, the voice or thought). You can respond that you believe that your clients have that experience. If questioned further, you can respond from a neutral exploratory inquisitive stance: "Why don't we check it out together?" "I'd be interested in finding out more about what you have found helpful and not so helpful in dealing with the (distressing) feelings you have during and after this experience. That way we can find coping strategies that work for you so you can get on with living your life and going for your goals."

It is important that you explore with your clients the physical sensations that often accompany emotions. For example, with fear there is often an increase in heart rate, jumpiness, or tightening of muscles. By helping your clients to notice the physical sensations that precede or accompany the identification of an emotion, their experience of the physical sensations is seen as "normal." You and your clients can then discuss ways that thoughts about physical sensations can serve to increase and/or decrease certain emotions.

Clinical Consideration: The Language You Use

Use of words and phrases like "we," "everyone," "all of us," and "many of us" in both individual and group therapy is more connecting, depathologizing, and destigmatizing. By using this type of inclusive language, a range of emotions, thoughts, and physical sensations are seen as part of being human rather than a sign that your clients are categorically different from others.

Acceptance and Willingness

A stance of increased acceptance of emotional experiences is implicit in the discussion and understanding of emotions and the ongoing normalization and validation process in therapy. *Acceptance* is defined as being open, receptive, and nonjudgmental about various aspects of our experience (Wilson & DuFrene, 2009). Paradoxically, trying to avoid or control unwanted thoughts or emotions can result in an increase in these thoughts or emotions, or increased energy spent on struggling with the thought or emotion (Leahy, Tirch, & Napolitano, 2011). Rather than focusing on often-ineffective control strategies to deal with emotions, encourage your clients to enhance understanding, acceptance, and coming into contact with a range of emotions. This focus on acceptance increases your clients' sense of self-efficacy while the associated willingness to experience affect enhances your clients' pursuit of their goals.

—EXERCISE: Pink Elephant

Ask your clients to think of a pink elephant for thirty seconds. Then ask them to imagine every aspect of the pink elephant. After thirty seconds, ask your clients to not think about pink elephants for the next two minutes. Discuss with your clients how this exercise went. Were they able to not think about pink elephants for two minutes? Use this exercise to highlight the difficulty with thought stopping and trying to control or avoid unwanted thoughts and associated feelings. Then discuss experiential acceptance.

Experiential acceptance provides another way to relate to private internal experiences and events. Instead of attempts at avoiding, controlling, or battling with distressing internal experiences, experiential acceptance enables us to come into contact with them and thereby continue to move in the direction of valued goals. By accepting difficult emotions and experiences, we acknowledge not only that distressing experiences are an inherent part of life but also that, by allowing these experiences, we can work toward our goals and create a more meaningful life. The goal of acceptance is not to rid ourselves of difficult thoughts, emotions, and experiences (an impossible goal to achieve!) but to live more consistently with our values and goals. And acceptance inherently involves self-acceptance, self-validation, and self-compassion. In the case of our clients, for example, instead of staying in bed to avoid suspicious or paranoid thoughts and the feelings associated with them, clients gradually move in valued directions by working toward their goals of getting out of bed and going to volunteer at the hospital. They are aided in this by enhanced emotion regulation strategies and the foundation of skills these strategies provide, as well as the practice of self-validation and self-compassion, all of which increase their ability to cope with distressing emotions and engage in exposure to feared situations and internal experiences.

Willingness ties acceptance with motivational engagement and committed action. By being willing to experience some upsetting feelings, clients can live a more value-consistent life and engage in committed action to work toward their goals. Willingness involves "doing what works," in spite of distressing emotions, in order to work toward living a more meaningful, goal-directed life.

Emotions are often tied to activities that we engage in to live consistently with our values and goals. For example, I may feel anxious about starting a volunteer position, as I don't feel very confident yet in social situations. However, no matter how well prepared I am or how confident I become, it may be necessary to feel some anxiety in order to begin volunteer work, and continue to work toward the goal of getting a paying job.

Clinical Tip

Your clients can become upset if they have a misconception about what is meant by acceptance. You will need to clearly define acceptance and to clarify any misunderstandings. Acceptance is not wishing for the emotions, experiences, symptoms, or illness. Nor is acceptance giving up. In fact, it is the opposite of giving up or resignation. Acceptance along with the willingness to experience difficult experiences enables clients to engage in avoided activities and work toward valued goals. Clients are doing the opposite of giving up or giving in. Furthermore, acceptance does not necessarily mean being happy about having an illness such as schizophrenia. In fact, we can have an illness or issues that we do not welcome or want to have but still accept that we have the illness and issues. Again we, as therapists, engage in a delicate dance with our clients. It is critical that we are able to empathize with our clients about distressing emotions, experiences, symptoms, and their illness(es). We may wish that our clients did not have "psychoses" or "schizophrenia" and yet also accept that our clients have distressing emotions, symptoms, and illness(es). Acceptance does not mean we don't want the best for our clients. Acceptance and willingness are some of many processes that can enable our clients to live more meaningful lives. This finding is critical to the research outcome choices made in CBTp. A focus on symptom levels (as compared to symptom distress or believability) as an outcome for CBTp may be misleading, since clients may report more symptoms due to more acceptance and less stigma associated with these symptoms.

It is important to link acceptance and willingness to engage in committed action with clients' personal values and goals. To increase motivation, highlight the connection between values and goals with willingness to engage in goal-directed activity. Form 6.4, Valued Activities, Willingness, Values, and Goals, is a helpful tool to make links between committed action and values and goals. This connection is particularly important as goal-directed activity often can involve coming into contact with distressing voices.

Mindfulness

Mindfulness is defined as moment to moment, nonjudgmental, present-centered awareness that is developed on purpose (Kabat-Zinn, 1990). The mindfulness process involves a nonjudgmental accepting of our internal and external experience. Therefore, mindfulness involves the process of coming into contact with distressing thoughts, delusions, feelings, experiences (such as hallucinations), and physical sensations. In mindfulness, the intention is for the clients (and therapist) to notice or observe experiences such as thoughts, emotions, and/or physical sensations and let them pass without judging or reacting to them. Mindfulness can enable exposure to distressing thoughts and experiences rather than the avoidance that is so often practiced and associated with "negative" or disturbing thoughts, delusions, and hallucinations. The present-moment awareness in mindfulness facilitates experiencing cognitions or thoughts as mental events that clients can "just" notice or observe; that is, through mindfulness practice and discussion or processing of the mindfulness experience, a more metacognitive and metaexperiential stance can be facilitated. *Metacognition,* or metathinking, involves exploring beliefs about thinking or thinking about thinking. Likewise, a *metaexperiential stance* toward emotions involves noticing our emotional schemas, or our philosophies or beliefs about emotions (Leahy et al., 2011). Thoughts can be viewed as "just thoughts" rather than automatically jumping to the conclusion that thoughts are facts. Instead of getting caught in, or reacting to, thoughts, delusions, images, and voices, one can "just" observe thoughts and experiences such as hallucinations.

Through mindfulness exercises (for example, noticing the busy nature of our minds or what we often refer to as "monkey mind") and the processing of mindfulness exercises in session, you can help to normalize distressing intrusive thoughts, upsetting emotions, and unusual perceptual experience. (See below for more on mindfulness exercises.) Your clients are able to become more aware and accepting of their full range of thoughts, emotions, sensations, images, sounds, and voices (either positive or negative). The normalization of the human experience of busy thoughts, self-talk, and a range of emotions and physical sensations can diminish client self-judgment and self-criticism. In addition, the normalization involved in discussing and processing mindfulness exercises can reduce the internalized self-stigma that is so often present in those who experience psychosis. Critically, present awareness provides an alternative process to the maladaptive processes of rumination and worry that so frequently accompany psychosis. Finally, mindfulness approaches allow for a reduction in distress and an enhanced ability to engage in meaningful activities and the pursuit of valued goals (Harris, 2009).

Mindfulness Exercises

Mindfulness encompasses both "formal" and "informal" exercises. Formal guided mindfulness exercises can be played on a CD or downloaded from the Internet (see our website, http://www

.treatingpsychosis.com). Below is a list of brief mindfulness exercises to develop formal and informal mindfulness practice:

- Mindful Breath

- Mindful Awakening

- Mindful Morning Body Scan

- Mindful Tasting, Eating, and Drinking

- Loving-Kindness Meditation

- Mindful Sounds

- Mindful Noting of Bodily Sensations

- Mindful Present Moment

- Mindful Declining

- Mindful Images

- Mindfulness of Self-Talk

- Mindfulness of Voices

(See our website http://www.treatingpsychosis.com for examples of these mindfulness approaches.)

Informal mindfulness approaches are shorter strategies that can be integrated throughout the day. Informal practices can be like "mini vacations" of awareness. Two such practices are three mindful breaths and mindfulness bells. (In mindfulness bells, preidentified cues—such as the color orange or going through a doorway—are used to remind one to engage in a short mindfulness practice.) Mindfulness exercises are practiced in and out of session during the therapy as well as (ideally) on an ongoing basis after therapy has finished. Collaboratively discuss and process client reactions to experiences of, and challenges with, doing each mindfulness exercise. Of course, this processing includes both in-session and between-session practice. It is important for you to emphasize that it often takes time to "get" mindfulness and to feel like one is benefiting from it. Like surfing, skateboarding, or skiing for the first time, one needs to proceed gently, keep practicing, and ride with the different experiences. Just as each wave is different, so is each mindfulness practice. And any and all practices are what they are—neither good nor bad. Again, as in an activity like surfing, clients may not notice quick progress, feel like they "get it," or benefit from the exercise at first. Perseverance is key!

Mindfulness approaches need to be tailored for those who experience psychosis (see Chadwick et al., 2005; 2009). Modifications for work with psychosis include, but are not limited to, an emphasis on assessment of appropriateness for practice given current symptoms, distress levels, ability to cope with affect, and overall functioning. It is important to engage in greater psychoeducation regarding the process of mindfulness and what to expect, normalize the ubiquity of distressing thoughts and experiences, provide more graded and shorter guided practices (say, a few minutes in duration), emphasize "informal" mindfulness practices, and increase time for you and your clients to process the experience and reinforce more adaptive shifts.

Clinical Tip

Many individuals find mindfulness very difficult to understand and/or do. Therapeutically, it can be beneficial to first introduce the concept of mindfulness along with some extremely brief, in-session mindfulness exercises, and to discuss these experiences in some depth before "assigning" mindfulness exercises between sessions. If clients are hesitant or don't want to do these exercises often, it is best to explore reasons and revisit this skill in a more limited manner, or at other times during the therapy. It is important not to force mindfulness. Many people will say things like "Oh, I tried that—that doesn't work for me" about relaxation, meditation, and/or mindfulness. Introducing it gradually and adjusting the pace as necessary may help clients who struggle with practice.

Clinical Consideration: Approach Mindfulness Slowly

Proceed slowly with these exercises. Start with very short, guided exercises using the breath or the different senses. Some individuals may experience psychotic symptoms, such as hearing a voice, when doing a mindfulness exercise. A reassuring, curious, and supportive tone can be helpful. For example, you might say, "Thank you for letting me know—we do expect that these types of experiences may come up," "Are you okay with discussing this experience a little further and seeing what we can learn from it?" or "Part of the purpose of these exercises is to notice a range of experiences without reacting to them."

When discussing mindfulness exercises with your clients and processing their experience with them, gentle reminders such as these can be helpful:

- Mindfulness is about allowing what is.

- Mindfulness is not the goal but part of the journey.

- Mindfulness is hard to do; distraction is a given.

- When distracted, gently return to the breath.

- If you notice your mind wandering, bring your awareness back gently, as gently as a feather falling on cotton balls.

- There is no such thing as a bad mindfulness exercise.

- Failure is impossible.

- We are building our mindfulness muscles—this does not happen overnight.

Compassion-Focused Approaches

Compassion-focused therapy approaches are an integral part of the treatment model and treatment approach. CFT strategies are incorporated throughout each session of the treatment as well as implicitly in the therapist stance within the treatment. CFT is a highly empathetic and caring approach to suffering that is well-suited to the harsh, critical, and often frightening experiences of paranoia and voices. In addition, CFT implicitly addresses the shame and self-stigma that frequently accompany a diagnosis of a schizophrenia-spectrum disorder. The research of Gilbert and colleagues (2001) indicates the importance of shame and self-criticism in maladaptive patterns of thought and behavior that maintain and exacerbate negative internal states such as psychosis. Through CFT approaches, your clients learn a range of techniques that facilitate an increased awareness of negative interactions with themselves, such as self-criticism. Over time, the blaming, self-critical stance toward oneself is substituted with an approach that emphasizes care for one's well-being and an increased stance toward self-understanding, empathy, and nonjudgment (Gilbert, 2009). CFT approaches are important as they dampen the activation of the threat emotion system while enhancing the affiliative/soothing emotion system, thereby increasing the ability for your clients to move in the direction of valued goals (the drive emotion system). Please see Gilbert's model of these emotion systems in figure 2.1 in chapter 2.

Similar to traditional CBT, CFT has at its core a compassionate therapeutic stance. CFT focuses on the development and enhancement of compassion for self and others. One example of a CFT strategy for those with psychosis is the development and use of the image of the "ideal nurturer" to counter the impact of denigrating hallucinations. A method that can be used for those who experience distressing delusions, such as others ridiculing them, is writing self-compassionate coping cards and/or self-compassionate letters. Other examples include the use of the two-chair technique to directly address the client's "inner bully" (see Gumley, Braehler, Laithwaite, MacBeth, & Gilbert, 2010; Braehler et al., 2013; Tai & Turkington, 2009).

Clinical Considerations: Preliminary Work for CFT

Clients who have a propensity to engage in self-criticism often find compassion-focused work foreign, challenging, and frightening (Gumley et al., 2010). Notably, a similar response is also typical for those who have trauma histories and are self-stigmatizing. It is critical that work is done first around decreasing fear or desensitizing distressing affect associated with compassion-focused work. Fears, apprehension, and attitudes toward compassion-focused work should be explored and addressed at the outset. In addition, emotional regulation strategies can be developed as a foundation to tolerate both positive and negative affect and the emotions generated in CFT. Techniques described by Linehan (1993), Leahy et al. (2011), and Khoury and Lecomte (2012) suggest how positive emotional experiences can be generated in therapy and used for emotional regulation.

Types of Compassion-Focused Exercises

Form 6.5 provides clinical CFT exercises such as those listed below. These types of CFT exercises should be integrated in each module to reinforce a compassionate stance toward self and others.

Compassionate intention

> Self: the intention to treat myself with loving-kindness and caring

> Others: the intention to treat others with compassion or caring

Compassionate attention

> Notice nature, compassionate acts, compassionate speech, and so on

Compassionate thoughts and compassionate reasoning

> Double standard: how would you think about the situation if a friend was experiencing it?

> Self-criticism versus constructive self-correction

> Compassionate approaches to self-shaming

Compassionate images

> Compassionate nurturer: try to generate an image of an ideal compassionate other

> Compassionate role models or mentors: identify a compassionate person or role model (for example, Mother Teresa, the Dalai Lama, Gandhi)

Compassionate behavior and acts

> Kindness to self and others

> How you would treat a friend

Compassionate coping cards—examples of themes for coping card statements (these should be written in your client's words):

> If my compassion does not include myself, it is not complete.

> I am deserving of compassion and caring.

Compassionate letter to self

Cognitive Flexibility: Cognitive Defusion and Cognitive Reappraisal

We discuss cognitive flexibility within the larger frame of psychological flexibility. Consistent with ACT, by enhancing cognitive flexibility and decreasing cognitive fusion, clients are freed up to work more toward valued life goals. It is important to address thoughts and thinking styles ("automatic thoughts") given the human tendency to have cognitive distortions, make cognitive errors, or have "hot" thoughts. For those with psychosis, there is an increased tendency to have particular types of cognitive biases or distortions (see Beck et al., 2009):

- Jumping to conclusions (more quickly and with less information than others; this tendency is heightened when stressed)

- An externalizing bias (blaming others)

- An intentionalizing bias (attributing negative or harmful intentions to others)

- An egocentric bias (a tendency to think the focus is on oneself)

- A self-serving bias (a tendency to think in ways that benefit oneself)

We incorporate cognitive reappraisal or cognitive restructuring as a process or approach that can be employed to notice thoughts aw well as gently consider alternative ways of understanding and thinking, thereby enhancing cognitive flexibility skills.

Clinical Consideration: Threat

For many clients who experience psychosis, it is not possible to engage in acceptance of distressing thoughts, delusions, and experiences such as voices, due to the veracity of their beliefs in the threat involved. Understandably, it is important to work with thoughts and beliefs around threat that increase experiential avoidance and thereby reinforce threat beliefs. For example, if clients hear voices that tell them that the CIA is wanting to harm their family, they would think that to reduce risk they would need to constantly scan for threats (that is, be hypervigilant) and respond as necessary to keep their family safe. Given the perceived threat, approaches such as mindfulness and acceptance would be very scary and deemed as unsafe. In order for these clients to engage in working toward valued goals, they would (understandably) need to ensure that their fears regarding risk or threat were not accurate. As Leahy and colleagues (2011) indicate, cognitions can have a mediating role in change—that is, a shift in cognitions may facilitate the occurrence of change. The processes involved in addressing threat and the veracity of beliefs and delusions is frequently complex and varies by individual. Strategies such as catch it, check it, change it (chapter 6); examining the evidence (chapter 8); behavioral experiments (chapter 8); the defense attorney technique for checking out evidence (chapter 8); exploring emotional reasoning (chapter 6); looking for alternative explanations through the use of a pie chart (chapter 8); and so on can be very helpful in chipping away at the thoughts and fears regarding imminent threat. In this case, cognitive reappraisal strategies can be used as part of the process of therapy to enhance cognitive defusion and increase our clients' ability to engage in therapeutic processes and strategies in order to work toward their goals. It is important to emphasize that cognitive reappraisal does not involve thought stopping or thought suppression, both of which are countertherapeutic. Rather, cognitive reappraisal is conducted to enhance the ability of our clients to engage in therapeutic and helpful processes that will enable them to work toward valued life goals.

The Thought Record, Thinking Styles, and "Catch It, Check It, Change It"

The use of a thought record is an extremely powerful tool to notice and track thinking or automatic thoughts. See the thought reords in Greenberger and Padesky (1995), Beck (1995), and Beck et al. (1979)—all are good examples. When using a thought record in treatment, it is important to start with a simplified version of the thought record—two columns with the event and then the thought. The thought record should be completed collaboratively in session with your clients to problem-solve any misunderstandings or confusion between emotions and thoughts. When using the thought record at home, your clients can look for changes in emotion and notice any thoughts that accompany these changes. Normalize that we all have a range of thoughts and thinking styles as well as distortions or biases in thinking. Clients may be hesitant to discuss certain thoughts that they may assume are nonnormative. For example, intrusive thoughts about hurting someone or intrusive sexual thoughts are common in the general population. Psychoeducation can help your clients be less preoccupied or worry less about particular thoughts. By normalizing, we also help our clients to use helpful rather than ineffective avoidant strategies in understanding and dealing with a range of emotions. (We also address intrusive thoughts as they relate to OCD in chapter 8 and our website http://www.treatingpsychosis.com.)

In the "catch it, check it, change it" approach, the "check it" part can involve a vast array of strategies (see thinking styles listed in form 6.6). The thinking styles form provides a list of common thinking "styles" or "traps" that can be reviewed with your client to discover any thinking styles that your client might be prone to. Ideally, ask your clients to read the list of thinking styles with you and see if they notice any that they use. If they use a particular thinking style, ask them, if possible, whether they can give a personal example. We also use this list when clients fill out a thought record. This helps clients to complete the thought record and notice their thinking styles.

We have found that using the 3Cs—catch it, check it, change it—for thoughts is a very powerful strategy for clients. The 3Cs help them to increasingly notice their thoughts, check out alternative understandings, and change the original thought(s) based on a more accurate or helpful way of thinking. We have added a fourth column and category to the 3Cs—which are now the 4Cs: catch it, check it, change it with compassion—that cues our clients to shift or change their thoughts in a compassionate way and treat themselves with compassion when engaging in this approach (see form 6.7).

Positive Emotions

As previously indicated, our treatment model involves a positive psychology–infused treatment approach that has at its core a focus on strengths and wellness. We address strengths, coping strategies, and resources throughout the treatment—in assessment, conceptualization, treatment planning, staying well, and each of the treatment sessions. Positive psychology is incorporated in each session, including the between-session practice review, as well as at the end of each session by focusing on accomplishments, strengths, efforts, and adaptive shifts. This positive psychology approach is foundational to the therapeutic stance and understanding of your clients. It is based on Seligman's (2002) work as well as the "broaden and build" theory of positive emotion (Fredrickson, 1998; 2001).

A positive emotion focus involves fostering positive experiences rather than suppressing or avoiding "negative" experiences. By enhancing the experience and encouragement of positive emotions, positive neurochemicals such as oxytocin and dopamine can be generated (Hanson, 2009). A focus on positive emotions can counter the negative (threat-based) bias of the brain. This enhances the brain's neuroplasticity so that (positive) "neurons that fire together, wire together." The development and enhancement of positive emotions is woven throughout the treatment. We have found that our clients gravitate toward certain practices (for example, gratitude and savoring) and with practice are increasingly able to incorporate these strategies in their day-to-day life. As with all of these approaches, we emphasize that these practices are like exercise—it takes time and repetition to get better at them and benefit from them.

Form 6.7 also presents a 3Cs for positive thoughts, images, and emotions. The 3Cs in this case involve (1) catching or creating the positive thought, image, or emotion; (2) cultivating and consolidating the thought, image, or emotion using the five senses and by prolonging the experience; and (3) connecting or linking the positive thought, image, or emotion with neutral and then with negative thoughts, images, emotions, or voices. Therefore, we work therapeutically on noticing, accepting, or shifting the relationship with distressing thoughts or experiences and noticing, creating, and enhancing positive thoughts and experiences.

Form 6.8 outlines a number of positive emotion exercises. These exercises, among others, help clients develop gratitude, remember positive memories and images, savor experiences, re-script their previous narrative or experiences, and use the breath. We highlight the importance of these "positive" approaches for neuroplasticity to decrease the negative bias and enhance the positive. See Hanson (2009; 2013) and http://www.treatingpsychosis.com for information on additional strategies for generating positive emotions and happiness as well as information on the burgeoning neuroscience behind these approaches. Hanson has also developed CDs on meditations for happiness that can be recommended or used with clients (see the Websites section in Resources).

Resilience

A resiliency-oriented focus is also implicit in the treatment approach. This approach involves using coping strategies, strengths, meaning, and values to adapt to adversity. According to the post-traumatic growth literature, resiliency is developed through attempting to find, and finding, meaning in adversity. As per Kent and Davis (2010), this involves a focus on the development and enhancement of positive emotions, an enhanced sense of control (developed through commitment and committed action and a shift to an internal locus of control), active coping, stress management and engagement, facing rather than avoiding fear or anxiety, enhancing cognitive flexibility, and finding meaning and value in adversity.

Committed Action to Valued Life Goals, Self-Care, and Health

Committed action to valued life goals includes a focus on self-care and health-enhancement strategies that deal with exercise, diet, sleep, smoking, and substance use. A number of health behaviors, self-care strategies, and coping strategies are essential to address in therapeutic work with those with psychosis. A survival analysis study of the entire Danish population found that the lifespan for adults with a diagnosis of schizophrenia was on average (tragically) shorter than those without a diagnosis of schizophrenia—18.7 years shorter for men and 16.3 years for women (Laursen, 2011). Of particular note, mortality due to physical diseases and medical conditions contributed to a much greater extent to the shortened lifespan than other causes such as accidents, suicide, or homicide. Laursen's findings point to the importance of addressing physical health conditions that can contribute to shortened lifespan (for example, weight gain associated with some antipsychotics, type 2 diabetes, and cardiovascular disease). These findings also highlight the potential sequelae of weight gain and the impact of the social determinants of health such as marginalization and poverty on our clients. A culturally informed and competent approach to treatment will not only recognize but also address these issues at the individual and societal level. We focus below on the importance of addressing health-related behaviors and issues such as exercise, diet, sleep, substance use, and smoking.

Exercise: Clinical trials have indicated that exercise can result in increases in brain volume in the hippocampus in individuals with a diagnosis of schizophrenia. Given that difficulties in learning and memory in schizophrenia are associated with smaller brain volume in the hippocampus (Alloway, 2011), exercise is an important goal to focus on. The benefits of exercise for enhancing mood and decreasing stress and symptoms of anxiety and depression have consistently been supported. (See Otto & Smits, 2011 for a resource on the benefits of exercise for mental health conditions.)

Diet: Given the above findings regarding life expectancy, weight gain associated with some antipsychotic medications, and the association of a poor diet with immune functioning and stress, psychoeducation about a healthy diet and exercise is of paramount importance. Additionally, engagement in problem solving regarding the cost of healthy eating is an important, yet challenging, focus in treatment, given the often-limited income of those with psychosis and the associated issues of social justice.

Sleep: Sleep difficulties can act as a trigger and maintaining factor for psychosis. Research has indicated that there is a strong association between insomnia and paranoia (Freeman et al., 2010; Freeman, 2011). Sleep interventions for sleep difficulties and insomnia typically involve psychoeducation, instructions in and application of sleep hygiene principles, stimulus control therapy, relaxation, cognitive restructuring, and addressing relapse. Research has found reduced rates of insomnia and of persecutory delusions as a result of interventions that address sleep hygiene (Myers, Startup, & Freeman, 2013). Given the weight gain that can be experienced by individuals on some antipsychotic medication, the increased incidence of sleep apnea associated with weight gain may need to be assessed and addressed. In addition, the incidence of trauma history in those with psychosis speaks to the importance of addressing the potential link of trauma with sleep disturbances.

Substance Use: Given the significantly higher rates of substance use in those with lived experience of psychosis, substance use is a critical area for intervention. The research literature indicates that an integrated approach to substance use and psychosis (wherein both the substance use and mental health issues are addressed by the same health care provider or team in the same setting) demonstrates the best outcomes. Motivational interviewing and strategies to enhance focus on valued goals that are inconsistent with substance use should be integrated throughout the treatment. When addressing helpful and unhelpful coping strategies, clients often identify substance use as an unhelpful coping strategy, which is then a focus for treatment. It is not possible to do justice here to the research literature in this area and the importance of addressing substance use in a collaborative, nonjudgmental, and goal-oriented manner. If substance use is an issue that gets in the way of clients working toward valued goals or is identified by your client as a focus for treatment or change, substance use should be an integral focus of the treatment in subsequent modules. Please see "Psychosis and Substance Use" in the Resources section for more information.

Smoking: Smoking cessation efforts as well as harm reduction approaches for smoking have received increased focus, given the much higher smoking rates in those with psychosis and the health sequelae of smoking. Please see "Smoking Cessation" in the Resources section for more information on this area.

Between-Session Practice

Collaboratively decide on the between-session practice, clarify understanding, and problem-solve any potential barriers to practice. Ask your clients to record their intention and commitment to the between-session practice on the Session Summary (form 5.1) and tie between-session practice with cues or daily activities such as meals, breaks, or a commitment to the times of the day to practice. (Watches, clocks, or cellular phones can be programmed to send reminders.) Sample handouts should be given to your clients, as well as the corresponding blank forms for them to fill out.

Feedback from Client on the Session

Solicit feedback from your clients during and at the end of each session as well as when processing emotion regulation exercises. Feedback increases collaboration and responsiveness on the part of the therapist, and helps to clarify any misunderstandings or concerns that can impact engagement, the therapeutic relationship, and emotion regulation.

Summary of Session

Ask your clients to read over the session handout at home and share this handout with family, friends, or caregivers, if they want to. Model a strengths-focused approach by asking clients to identify one personal strength, quality, or accomplishment from the session. If your clients find it difficult to do so, you can cue with examples you have noticed or ask what a friend or family member might say. This reinforces your client's efforts, strengths, accomplishments, and progress, and introduces the coping or grounding exercise.

Coping Exercise (Optional)

See form 4.2 in the appendix for a selection of coping exercises.

Additional Resources

For more information, please see the Resources section of this book. You will find many of the forms in the appendix; they are also available for download at http://www.newharbinger.com/24076. (See the back of this book for instructions on how to access them.) Additional materials not available in this book can be found on our website at http://www.treatingpsychosis.com.

CHAPTER 7

Module 4: Action Toward Valued Goals: Overcoming Barriers to Value-Consistent Living

In this module, we address some of the barriers to working toward valued goals. These include low motivation, low energy, and defeatist beliefs. In particular, negative symptoms in psychosis are addressed to facilitate clients moving in the direction of their valued goals—that is, negative symptoms are addressed as part of the process of overcoming barriers to living a value-consistent life and achieving valued goals. We incorporate behavioral activation, including the importance of work with values, to facilitate getting active and achieving goals. Material and processes addressed can be covered in approximately three to five sessions, based on the individual needs of your client.

Materials

See appendix for forms. They are also available for download at http://www.newharbinger.com/24076. (See the back of this book for instructions on how to access them.)

Modifications for Group Interventions

The content and strategies in this module are amenable to modification for group interventions. Group process can enhance motivation and encourage work toward valued goals. Positive peer pressure and review of between-session practice can increase committed action and engagement. Motivation can also be enhanced by placing group members' values and goals on a poster on the wall in the group room. In addition, the development of group values and goals can enhance the group's movement in valued directions and a sense of a collective momentum and goals. A range of motivational levels of group members can be helpful to enhance modeling of activation and to instill hope and possibility. A group motto such as "Go in the direction of your hopes, not your fears" can also enhance a shared vision. Defeatist beliefs, so common in those with psychosis, can be addressed and explored in the group context, and increased perspective can be generated by group members providing feedback to one another as well as recounting and reinforcing accomplishments and successes.

Goals and Outline of Module (3 to 5 sessions)

This module focuses on committed action by addressing barriers to goal-directed activity, such as negative symptoms. Therapeutic strategies focus on enhancing motivation through behavioral activation strategies and getting active in order to be able to work toward valued goals. This module flows from the work on values identification in module 2 (see chapter 5). Emotion regulation skills, a focus of module 3 (see chapter 6) are also important here; they provide your client with ways to cope with distressing emotions or symptoms that may arise as a result of behavioral activation and working toward goals. In addition, emotion regulation skills were developed to enhance client efficacy in order that clients decrease their experiential avoidance (for example, staying at home to not hear voices) and increase committed action toward valued life goals.

Overview of Treatment Area for Clinician

Subsequent to the stabilizing and foundational therapeutic work on emotion regulation and resilience, the therapy focuses on moving in the direction of valued goals. Negative symptoms (often defined as deficits in motivation, speech, emotion, and pleasure) are addressed next in the therapeutic process and throughout therapy as required to enhance motivation, engagement in therapy, and work toward valued goals. Unfortunately, negative symptoms are often given less emphasis in the treatment of those who experience psychosis than the more noticeable positive symptoms (such as hallucinations and delusions). However, the importance of recognizing and addressing negative symptoms and other barriers to goal achievment is essential, and should be a key focus initiated early in therapy and actively maintained throughout treatment. Indeed, data have suggested that negative symptoms may have a more detrimental impact on functioning, prognosis, and overall quality of life than positive symptoms (Rabinowitz, De Smedt, Harvey, & Davidson, 2002) and that, along with cognitive function, negative symptom severity is among the most powerful predictors of general community functioning and adaptation (Wittorf, Wiedemann, Buchkremer, & Klingberg, 2007). With these compelling findings in mind, interventions specifically targeting negative symptoms are a critical component in therapy for individuals experiencing psychosis. Unfortunately, there is also a relative lack of empirically validated treatments available to address negative symptoms as compared to positive symptoms. Consistent with our model, we integrate an understanding of the causes and roles of negative symptoms as well as work on values and committed action toward valued goals.

Barriers to Activation: Defeatist Beliefs, Stigma, and Low Cognitive Confidence

Negative symptoms and other barriers to action have been found to be associated with "defeatist beliefs" regarding predicted enjoyment and mastery of activities. However, research indicates that pleasure ratings for activities are similar between those with and without psychosis, but those with psychosis are not able to sustain the experience of pleasure for as long as others. Mastery or the ability to complete an activity successfully is underestimated by those with psychosis, which can hamper engagement in meaningful activities.

Defeatist beliefs will be voiced frequently during activity scheduling sessions. Therefore, behavioral experiments to predict mastery and pleasure can be extremely helpful. Using a rating of 0–10 helps your clients notice small changes and develop greater skill in making finer or more granulated differentiations around emotions such as pleasure. You can start first by using evidence of behaviors successfully achieved (coming to the therapy session) and enjoyed (for example, time with family). It is important to discuss avoidance and the paradoxical short-term success of avoidance as a way of coping with severe anxiety or an extreme experience of psychosis. If a positive log is taken, it might show periods of time thinking, watching TV, listening to the radio, and making efforts to cope with disturbing experiences. These can be reframed as heroic successes or at least courageous attempts to manage. Could we as clinicians really cope any better if we were in the client's shoes? Often there is an image that is linked to defeatist beliefs. One patient, Mary, said that, whenever she tried to do anything, she had an image of herself in an "asylum" corridor pleading for leave and her plea being firmly declined by her physician. Further exploration of the image revealed that, at that time, she herself felt too unwell for leave and that she actually appreciated the kindness of her physician. She could then replace the image of defeat with another image of the same clinician warmly praising her for her progress. Such schema-focused approaches can be used to moderate the defeatist beliefs that mediate many negative symptoms.

The metabelief of "my brain is broken" relates to the concept of cognitive confidence. Beliefs such as "I am able to converse," "I am able to be a friend," "My memory works reasonably well," and "I am able to think and problem solve" are all statements of cognitive confidence. Stigma often leads clients to believe that they cannot do many of the things these statements describe because their brains are "broken." And, unfortunately, mental health services can at times "collude" with this very stigmatizing view of psychosis and schizophrenia. Patients are often so stigmatized by the label of schizophrenia that they can simply give up. Destigmatizing approaches based on normalizing and an empowering attitude toward prognosis and how long medication will be taken can greatly help to improve clients' cognitive confidence and help negative symptoms.

Avoidance, Safety Behaviors, and Skill Development

In addition, those with lived experience of psychosis may not engage in certain activities due to avoidance or acquired "safety behaviors." Fears of the activation of voices or distressing thoughts and delusions can hamper involvement in social and other meaningful activities. Psychoeducation around avoidance, as well as a graded approach to behavioral activation, can address these fears. Through exposure or behavioral activation, your client can enhance distress tolerance skills associated with symptoms as well as learn that exposure to voices or distressing thoughts and delusions can enhance self-efficacy and pursuit of meaningful goals. A focus on social and other skill development can enhance competence and confidence. In addition, exercises that emphasize the development of the ability to maintain pleasurable experiences ("savoring," as mentioned in chapter 6) can be helpful to sustain enjoyable experiences.

Rationale for Behavioral Activation

Behavioral activation is a complementary approach that we use to work on "defeatist" beliefs. We emphasize behavioral activation (an approach initially developed for use with depression) to address barriers to working toward valued goals and a more meaningful life. Consistent with our treatment model and approach, behavioral activation is a practical therapeutic tool that maintains a core focus on understanding and identifying your clients' values in life and taking tangible steps in valued directions.

Although mood and psychotic disorders are generally held to be distinct syndromes, there is reasonable cause to believe that the psychotherapeutic interventions we use for depression may also be of benefit in treating negative symptoms. At a fundamental level, both conditions are marked by many similar subjective experiences, emotional states, and behavioral patterns. An examination of the shared experiences and symptoms and corresponding psychotherapeutic solutions suggests significant potential for finding tools to assist individuals experiencing negative symptoms.

Those who experience psychosis and negative symptoms often report (1) very low feelings of self-efficacy, (2) profound feelings of isolation, (3) lack of interest in activities, (4) thoughts around being a failure, (5) negative expectancies regarding themselves and their futures, and (6) suicidal thoughts (Beck et al., 2009). These symptoms are remarkably parallel to the core experiences routinely assessed for, and endorsed by, individuals experiencing depressive disorders, and negative symptoms routinely prove extremely challenging to distinguish from those of a comorbid mood or anxiety disorder (Beck et al., 2009). Also, affective blunting and affective incongruity can mask coexisting depression.

Negative symptoms, in the same manner as depression, typically involve patterns of behavior that lead to an increasingly vicious cycle of separation from sources of reinforcement and/or valued activity in people's lives. As people withdraw from engagement with their environment emotionally, cognitively, and behaviorally, the available sources of "reward" dwindle along with the capacity to find such experiences rewarding.

Using behavioral modification to reconnect with sources of positive reinforcement and personal value and meaning is the core aim driving behavioral activation (Hopko, Lejuez, Ruggiero, & Eifert, 2003). With this aim in mind, we integrate behavioral activation strategies as key clinical tools in helping individuals to address negative symptoms. Successfully helping clients to cope with the negative symptoms often associated with psychosis is a core element of therapy, both at the beginning of therapy work and throughout treatment. Behavioral activation strategies to enhance motivation, engagement, and work toward valued goals are key components of the treatment. In using behavioral activation, you and your clients will work to discover how they spend their time in day-to-day life and to begin drawing connections among emotions, activities, and the valued directions that your clients identify with. Using this information, your clients will be in a position to begin the gradual, but critical, process of reclaiming a sense of meaning, accomplishment, and enjoyment in life.

Agenda for Each Session

As in past sessions, you and your clients will begin by discussing the agenda. Collaboratively decide on the content and skills to be covered in the session, including time for check-in and any issues that may have arisen between sessions. It will be critical to focus your agenda on the review and troubleshooting of between-session practice. Any issues that have arisen can be placed on the session agenda and may be linked to its topic and content—for example, using activation targets to assist in a problem-solving process for a particular dilemma.

Check-In

You may start by completing a check-in with your clients based on their functioning since the last session, including the day of the current session. We have added a rating on motivation for use, if clinically appropriate. As in the previous module, the check-in can involve any of the ratings that follow.

Mood rating 0–10 (10 being the highest level of positive mood)

Anxiety rating 0–10 (10 being the highest level of anxiety)

Self-efficacy or accomplishment rating 0–10 (10 being the highest level of self-efficacy)

Psychosis rating 0–10 (10 constituting the highest level of distress associated with thoughts, delusions, and/or hallucinations such as voices)

Motivation rating 0–10 (10 constituting the highest level of motivation)

Summary and Link to Previous Chapter/Session

Discuss what your clients recall from the last session. Summarize material from the previous section, perhaps highlighting those areas in which your clients have noted concerns like withdrawal, low mood, low motivation, and/or low activity levels. You can suggest that the current topic may provide a useful way to help with these difficulties.

Review and Problem Solving of Between-Session Practice

Review of between-session practice is especially critical in this module. Ask about client experience with the planned activities from your last session. Once this module is underway, a review of activity and emotion tracking, along with a discussion of successes or difficulties in achieving activation goals, will form a large component of the sessions and approaches. In many ways, a behavioral activation session such as this one is structured entirely around processing, problem-solving, and modifying between-session practices.

Coping Exercise

See form 4.2, Coping Exercises.

Overview of Session/Topic Area for Clients

The overview includes psychoeducation. Discuss information about negative symptoms with your clients (see "Therapeutic Strategies and Exercises" below). Be sure to address client understanding of how defeatist beliefs and negative symptoms can get in the way of pursuing valued life goals. The behavioral activation topic can be introduced by noting any difficulties your clients have previously expressed regarding withdrawal, lack of enjoyment, lack of meaning, or other negative symptoms. Share with your clients that there is a connection between how we feel and what we are doing, and that an exploration of these patterns, with gradual adjustments to behaviors, may be useful in changing this cycle.

Clinician Stance

Your stance should emphasize normalization and empowerment, while at the same time using curiosity and inquisitiveness to provide a gentle "nudge" that may help encourage your clients to try new behavioral goals. Explain that even when we are sleeping or resting, we are always doing something. The question is whether we have some success in doing it and how much we enjoy it.

Therapeutic Strategies and Exercises

Collaboratively discuss barriers to committed action, including motivation, energy, or "negative symptoms" and the role of defeatist beliefs or thoughts. Discuss the information below with your clients.

Barriers to Action?

"Negative symptoms": *Negative symptoms* are thoughts, feelings, behaviors, or experiences that we don't experience or that we don't experience as much as others—or as much as we would like! Negative symptoms can involve a lack of energy, motivation, or interest. Other examples are not having much interest or pleasure in things, feeling little or no emotion, feeling like our emotions are dulled, and not doing certain activities such as day-to-day tasks, socializing, or going out with friends. When we have "negative symptoms," it can be hard to get active and do things—even things we usually enjoy!

Avoiding things: Sometimes we aren't active because we're avoiding something. For example, we might avoid going out in public because we feel anxious in social situations or we're afraid that we might have a bad experience. We all avoid some things, some of the time!

What happens when we avoid things?: While avoiding certain things may help us feel less anxious or less afraid in the short term, it can create problems in the long run. It can make it harder and harder to face the very things that we are avoiding. For this reason, it is important to work gradually toward being able to face those things that make us anxious or afraid.

Helpful Thoughts for Action

Thoughts, beliefs, assumptions, rules, or images can serve as barriers to goal-directed activity. As a result, it is important to first address these types of barriers or roadblocks to action. Form 7.1, ABC for

Action, provides a framework for exploring these barriers with your clients. First, complete the ABC for Action form with your client collaboratively in session. Then, if appropriate, ask your client to complete it for between-session practice. Begin by discussing the role of defeatist beliefs or other thoughts that can get in the way of us going for our goals. Ask your clients to try to notice thoughts that might get in the way of being more active. Remind your clients about the important role of values and meaningful goals in increasing motivation. After completing the inaction belief example or unhelpful thoughts example in form 7.1, ask your client to come up with a more helpful or balanced thought about the activity. When completing the form together, explore how the more helpful thought for getting active impacts both the emotional and behavioral consequences.

Behavioral Activation

Having addressed barriers to working toward goals—including thoughts, beliefs, assumptions, rules, or images that get in the way of goal-directed action—begin to discuss behavioral activation with your client. Talk about the steps in behavioral activation:

1. Record activities and emotions.

2. Identify values and valued life goals.

3. Choose valued activities.

4. Complete the valued activity ladder.

5. Plan activities and weekly targets.

1. Record Activities and Emotions

The core strategy at the beginning of most behavioral activation interventions is to ask your clients to record their activities, along with a rating for that time period using a scale you have mutually chosen. (See form 7.2 for one such record.)

Recording activities can look deceptively simple, but it forms the foundation of future activation work. With this tool, clinicians can accomplish several aims:

• Obtain a baseline of current activity levels.

• Identify recurrent patterns in clients' behaviors and emotions.

• Illustrate the two-way connection between behavior and emotion.

• Identify areas of strength to amplify.

- Understand the variety (or lack thereof) of current activities of clients.

- Understand the range of emotional experiences of clients.

- Gain a more concrete picture of how activities might be moving your client toward, or away from, valued areas in life.

Complete the Activity Form (form 7.2) with your clients. In addition to the activity, clients can record their emotion and sense of mastery experienced during the activity. A basic emotion scale can be a 0 to 10 rating, where 0 is "unhappy" or "withdrawn" and 10 is "happy" or "engaged.") However, use considerable flexibility in choosing an emotion or feeling that will best capture your clients' experience. Along with (or instead of) ratings of the emotion of happiness or engagement, you may ask your clients to record the degree to which they feel enjoyment or pleasure, and the degree to which they feel a sense of mastery, accomplishment, success, and/or achievement while completing the activity.

Clinical Tip

Activity and emotion recording might be a tough sell for some clients as it can be time intensive and may feel unnatural at first. Explore the potential benefits with your clients, both before and after using the strategy. Start first by completing an activity form together in session based on the day before and the day of your appointment. At this stage, it is very common for clients to assert that they do not have "any" accomplishments to note; however, this can be an ideal time to point out that even seemingly trivial things, such as getting out of bed or coming to the appointment, are accomplishments that move them toward their valued goals.

Once you and your client have completed an activity form in session, discuss completing an activity form for between-session practice. For many clients, it can be helpful to initially suggest recording activities for only one or two activities or for a day or two before attempting to record a full week of activities. From a motivation perspective, it may also be helpful to discuss with your clients writing down a core value, goal, or theme that they would like to emphasize during activities for the week on the activity form. If your clients complete the activity form in between sessions, process how it was for them, including any insights and difficulties encountered.

A side note for clinicians: if you haven't already, it might be helpful to try activity recording *yourself* for a week (or more) before suggesting it. Complete the Activity Form (form 7.2) yourself. This will help you gain an appreciation of the challenges and rewards it can present!

2. Identify Values and Valued Life Goals

As discussed throughout this book, the identification of valued life directions is a core guide for treatment overall, and it is particularly germane in a discussion of behavioral activation. Values can be presented as a "compass" to guide activation targets and behavioral goals. Again, it is important to highlight the distinction between a "value" and a "goal," as described in module 2 in chapter 5 (and see

Hayes et al., 1999 for more information). A *value* is a direction in which we are headed, while a *goal* is a specific objective we reach along the way. We never fully "reach" a value, but rather perpetually move toward it; therefore, values provide us with reliable and ongoing sources of motivation as well as information regarding which actions we might take next.

Your clients can begin by selecting three to five values that they identified in module 2 (chapter 5) as most important to them. While the most critical factor is that these values be truly your clients' (and not those you wish for your clients), you may gently encourage your clients to select areas that will increase variety in potential activity choices. For example, we often see clients who state their values in ways such as "be a better parent," "be a better friend," "be a better citizen." While these are all very noble aims, they *may* also suggest that the clients are underattending to their own needs. Collaboratively explore these areas with your clients, and, if appropriate, suggest the possibility of including an area such as "having fun."

Examples of values include:

- Being helpful to others

- Being compassionate to myself

- Being compassionate to others

- Being active

- Being healthy

It is important to reinforce and integrate values in the role of supporting valued activities and goals. In addition to listing values on the Values and Valued Activities form (7.3), you may suggest to your clients, as mentioned above, that they record values on their Activity Form (7.2). In addition, ask your clients to keep a copy of their values list on a coping card. (It may also be helpful to keep a copy of your clients' values list for your reference.)

3. Choose Valued Activities

Once values have been identified, you and your clients can collaboratively brainstorm potential activities that will help them to move in these valued directions. Use form 7.3 to record multiple values and associated valued activities generated by your client in session. Alternatively, a separate list can be made for each value and valued activities involved in working toward valued goals (see form 7.3). A core feature of appropriate ideas for valued activities is that, as behavioral targets, they should be observable, measureable, specific, and, to the degree possible, within the person's ability to complete.

Guidelines: Generating Ideas for Valued Activities

When generating ideas for valued activities, several guidelines can be kept in mind that will increase the likelihood of future success:

Identify activities for valued directions: Initially, a discussion of potential valued activities may lead to very broad, vague aims. Most people understandably want to "feel better" rather than get mired in the details of how to get there. Targets such as "feel happiness again," "get in shape," "get rid of my voices," or get a "boy/girlfriend" are too broad for use in activity lists. In these instances, it is important to identify what sort of activities would be involved in working toward these valued directions.

Identify small, digestible steps: Clients will often provide ideas in the form of broader goals they have; for example, a person who values education may suggest "finish high school" as an aim. While such targets are important sources of information, it is the small, digestible steps to complete that are most important to identify.

Collaboratively choose targets within clients' control: Quite frequently, clients and clinicians will also identify seemingly well-framed targets that inadvertently rely on factors outside of the individual's control. For example, an aim to "enjoy a conversation with a friend over coffee" may appear to fit the bill perfectly for someone valuing social connection. However, such a target is reliant on a number of extraneous factors: What if the friend is in a bad mood? Perhaps the friend will be perpetually busy. Maybe the friend doesn't like being in public. Instead, collaboratively choose targets that your client can take ownership of and plan in advance, therefore increasing chances of success. In this instance, "invite my friend to go for coffee" is an activity that can be much more reliably carried out.

Throughout the exploration of potential activity targets, it is critical to bear in mind that the most suitable activity ideas are not goals in and of themselves, but rather actions or behaviors that will increase the likelihood of achieving one's goal (Hayes et al., 1999). In the example above, the invitation is a specific, concrete, defined step that may assist one in moving toward a goal of establishing a regular friendship connection, all in the service of valuing one's social life. If the friend accepts the offer and the coffee meeting goes well, this provides natural reinforcement for the initial activity of extending the invitation. Should the outcome not be as hoped, it provides solid information to be used in problem solving during session; and, at the same time, your client can still find reinforcement in knowing that he or she is acting more in accord with personal values.

Generating activity ideas can also be a very healing exercise in its own right, as it often helps clients to realize that there are, in fact, a number of things they are capable of doing as they are. This is often a difficult notion for clients to recognize. One of the more helpful strategies in helping to generate ideas and gain benefit from the exercise can be to highlight those steps your clients have *already* taken without necessarily having realized it. You may choose to point out occasions you are already familiar with where your clients have taken action in accord with their values. If appropriate, you can even point out their attendance at the current appointment and ask, "What is important to you that allowed you to take this step?" By genuinely recognizing and applauding the efforts and achievements already made, you can facilitate the process of generating further ideas.

4. Complete the Valued Activity Ladder

For this section, please see the Activity Ladder (form 7.5). Some actions are more easily performed than others. For nearly all people, the notion of "becoming more social," "being a better son," or "getting an education" may sound appealing, but can quickly become overwhelming. The increased tendency to feel overwhelmed or defeated is a common underlying factor in negative symptoms, for those who experience them. By taking gradual, *concrete* steps in the directions of their life goals and values, our clients can begin to realize the behavioral changes that will help to lessen the impact of negative symptoms and to reclaim sources of enjoyment and meaning.

For each of the three to five identified values (see chapter 5 and form 5.2 for identified values), select approximately five activities from the brainstorming exercise that your client could feasibly perform. As noted above, aim for activities that can be planned in advance (to the degree possible). Also, choose a large majority of activities that can easily be repeated. While there is no harm from a few "one-offs," the ideal list will be comprised mainly of activities that can be used and reused, offering continuing opportunities for modification and reinforcement.

Once you and your clients have identified a set of activities for each value, it is time to arrange them into a "step-wise list" or ladder of activities, as shown in form 7.5. Complete the ladder of activities together with your clients. If you have previously used exposure hierarchies in the behavioral treatment of anxiety, this ladder will look somewhat familiar to you. Your clients should select a range of activities from comparatively easy to quite challenging for the ladder.

For some clients, it may be best to take an assortment of activities from the various valued directions they have identified and create one primary list. While there is no perfect number, selecting approximately seven to ten activities can be a good place to start. Alternately, you and your clients may choose to create a smaller list for each chosen value.

For each activity, your clients should assign a rating of how difficult they expect the task would be. This rating can be rank ordered based on the number of items in the ladder, or it can be done on a 0 to 10 scale, where 0 is "no avoidance, no difficulty" and 10 is "total avoidance, extreme difficulty." When arranging the ladder, it can be helpful to keep these points in mind:

- Aim for a range of difficulties. It can be helpful to have clients begin by rating a few items, and then insert further items as "tiebreakers." Ideally, there will be a full range across the scale.

- Seeing the growing hierarchy can be daunting. Reassure clients that, by placing an activity on the ladder or hierarchy, they are not binding themselves into doing it; rather, it is just another idea for future consideration in working toward their goals. For some clients, it may be helpful to include a few extra activities that they are already performing and wish to continue, now with the added explicit connection with their values.

- Activities can serve more than one value at a time. Such items may be particularly useful for inclusion in the ladder.

- Encourage selection of items that are more likely to be naturally and immediately reinforcing, particularly for the "easier" targets. Seeing tangible evidence of progress early on will help build momentum.

- While some clients may feel overwhelmed, others will quickly become self-critical and belittle their own efforts by noting how "insignificant" their planned activities may seem. It is important to stress to clients that the focus is on the movement they are making in the service of their values rather than on the perceived "magnitude" (or lack thereof) of the achievements on their lists.

5. Plan Activities and Weekly Targets

When the ladder is completed, the next step is to select one or two activities to target in the upcoming week, beginning with those rated as least difficult or least avoided. Having selected these activities, develop a concrete plan about their completion. When will they be completed? How long will your client spend on the activity? How many times will your client complete it during the week?

Scheduling the activities and recording their completion can be done in a number of different ways. If your clients have had success in using activity and emotion recording with form 7.2, encourage them to place the activity directly on the Activity Form (7.2) to complete later in the week. You may also choose to use the Emotion and Mastery Form (7.4) to plan the activities in a separate place. On this sheet, record the activity and note when it is to be completed and/or the number of times your clients will do the activity. It may also be helpful to include a core value, goal, or theme for the week that clients would like to emphasize throughout their activities.

It can also be very useful to use planned activities as an opportunity to test predictions about how difficult the activity will be and how it will impact on emotions. While planning in session, ask clients to rate their expected emotion and difficulty levels for each activity from 0 to 10 on the Emotion and Mastery Form (7.4), then rerate once the activity is actually completed. Such an exercise can provide a valuable way for clients to help counter the inertia they may be experiencing. In a similar vein, you may wish to note a core theme, goal, or value for each week as an incentive and reminder of the overall "why" behind the activities planned.

Allow for considerable latitude in planning exactly *how* the activity will be completed. For many individuals experiencing psychosis, these first steps may be fraught with especially high levels of self-doubt, fear, and negative expectations. Support your clients with appropriate guidance, while allowing them to also build a foundation of self-efficacy. Clients may also return having completed an activity that is different from what was planned; for example, going to a movie with a friend may have turned into a quiet night of board games if other symptoms were making a public event simply too overwhelming. At such times, remind your client (and yourself) of the fundamental aim: reconnecting with valued life directions. If this quiet game of checkers helped move your client toward strengthening friendships in the same way a movie date was originally intended, congratulate your client on a job well done.

Overcoming Barriers to Activation

It is to be expected that many clients will not complete all planned activities each week. Processing the barriers and difficulties that have arisen will form the foundation for practice of problem-solving skills, creativity, and new activity plans.

Problem-Solving Difficulties with Activation

Kanter, Busch, and Rusch (2009) highlight a useful framework for problem-solving difficulties with activation. Using a framework based in functional analysis, they distinguish between difficulties that arise in the antecedent or "setting the stage" phase of behavior, those to be found in the behavior or activity itself, and those that are based in the consequences of completing the behavior. When teaming with your client to problem-solve why a target behavior was not completed, it can be helpful to think in terms of barriers that can arise at the various phases: antecedent ("setting the stage"), activity/behavior, or consequence. See a list of potential areas to explore below:

- Is your client letting him- or herself off the hook with permission-giving thoughts?

- Did your client forget to do the behavior?

- Is your client remembering at the "wrong" time (for example, remembering to cook dinner while at work)?

- Does your client have enough time to do the activity?

- Are the necessary tools or equipment available?

- Does your client know how to complete the activity?

- Could it help to practice the activity in session?

- Did your client have difficulties completing the activity itself?

- Are other symptoms interfering with the activity?

- Are there barriers that arise as a consequence of completing the activity?

- Does the activity make the client feel uncomfortable afterward?

- Is there fear of higher expectations from others if your client is successful?

- Are others reacting poorly to the activity?

- Is there too little immediate reinforcement?

- Does your client have difficulty remembering the critical activity-value connection?

Clinical Considerations: Client Support

If available, significant others can be a tremendous boon in helping clients to reach their activation targets. On a broader level, simply sharing the practice exercises (form 7.2) with a supportive person can make a tremendous difference in increasing the likelihood of completing the activity. Lejuez, Hopko, Acierno, Daughters, and Pagoto (2011) also make use of a more specific behavioral "contracting." Simply put, *contracting* involves you and your clients identifying specific individuals and a few defined ways in which these people can assist your clients in meeting their behavioral goals. Not only is there benefit from making a "public commitment," but individuals in your clients' lives may finally see a more tangible opportunity to assist with specific behavioral goals. Additionally, the added benefit of strengthening interpersonal connections cannot be overstated.

Between-Session Practice

As noted above, sessions in this activation module are structured with the troubleshooting, processing, and planning of between-session practice as an explicit focus. Your between-session practice plan for the week will flow naturally from this discussion.

Feedback from Client on the Session

Ask your client for constructive feedback on the session. These questions can help solicit both positive and constructive feedback:

- What was most helpful today (or in this session)?

- What was least helpful?

- Are our activation targets a good fit for your values or what is important to you?

- Do our activation targets seem realistic for the time until our next session?

Summary of Session

Summarize the session for your clients and provide a written summary of this material (form 4.3). During the behavioral activation module, use this summary as another opportunity to highlight for your clients the connections among their values, their behavioral choices, and the way they are feeling. You may also emphasize your clients' courage, progress, and perseverance in their efforts to take concrete steps that will move them toward their valued goals. As always, be sure to reinforce your clients' openness to challenges, strong efforts, strengths, and accomplishments.

Coping Exercise

See form 4.2 in the appendix for examples.

Additional Resources

For more information, please see the "Resources" section of this book. You will find many of the forms in the appendix; they are also available for download at http://www.newharbinger.com/24076. (See the back of this book for instructions on how to access them.) Additional materials not available in this book can be found on our website at http://www.treatingpsychosis.com.

CHAPTER 8

Module 5: Understanding, Assessing, and Treating Distressing Thoughts and Delusions

In this module, we describe understanding, assessing, and treating distressing thoughts and delusions. A respectful and normalizing approach to work with distressing thoughts and delusions increases engagement, therapeutic exploration, and work toward valued goals. Consistent with our model, specific thoughts and delusions are explored and addressed with the goal of reducing distress and assisting client movement toward value-consistent living and valued goals. In this chapter, we build on the therapeutic work with thoughts, emotions, and behaviors from the modules on emotion regulation and behavioral activation, and complement these therapeutic approaches with a focus on additional therapeutic strategies such as metacognitive strategies, mindful compassion strategies, and behavioral experiments.

Materials

See the appendix for forms. They are also available for download at http://www.newharbinger. com/24076. (See the back of this book for instructions on how to access them.) Because the cognitive abilities and needs of clients vary, we've provided additional versions of some forms in this chapter on the New Harbinger website.

Modifications for Group Implementation

Group approaches to working with distressing thoughts and delusions proceed in a graded fashion by first engaging in psychoeducation and normalizatuion by discussing common thinking styles (see form 6.6 on thinking styles). Discussion of content typically starts with types of thinking styles that can be common—such as jumping to conclusions or catastrophizing—rather than moving directly into emotionally activating work with delusions. Terms such as "helpful" or "ways of thinking about a situation" can be used to enhance cognitive flexibility and defusion.

Clients typically find this graded approach respectful and depathologizing. The opportunity to share thoughts and experiences with others is inherently connecting and speaks to the common experience of distressing and intrusive thoughts, "monkey" mind, and critical self-talk. While enhancing their understanding of the lived experience of another, clients can also gently help one another to work toward more helpful and healthy ways of thinking about themselves and others. The group can be experienced as a place of support and growth and can serve to enhance empathy and theory of mind skills.

Clients and clinicians often fear reinforcement of, or "collusion" with, delusional beliefs, or that group members will give other members ideas that feed into their existing distressing thoughts or delusions. Taking a curious stance of checking out or exploring thoughts and thinking of thoughts as guesses rather than facts can be modeled and reinforced in the group. Clients share their experience at a pace that they determine. Some clients may be hesitant and feel anxious sharing in group and may become emotionally activated when discussing distressing thoughts and beliefs. It can be helpful for the leader at these points to remind group members that therapy work can, at times, involve feeling more anxiety as we are addressing important personal issues. Reinforcement of the use of grounding approaches and emotion regulation strategies is important at these times. Group leaders can guide the group in a coping exercise that is deactivating. Alternatively, group leaders can assist an individual client in session or by taking the client to a quieter room and returning when the group member is feeling less activated. Of course, activation of affect will have been addressed in the pregroup assessment, when establishing group guidelines, and in the emotion regulation strategies that form the foundation for therapy. Group discussion often highlights the common experience of unwanted or intrusive thoughts of a religious, sexual, aggressive, or other nature. Upon exploration with group members, links can often be made between intrusive thoughts and fears around mind reading (for example, "What if someone knew I had these thoughts?") or thought insertion (for example, "I don't think that way—someone must have put those thoughts in my head"). Asking for a show of hands around intrusive thoughts and normalizing the frequency of intrusive thoughts can be experienced as reassuring and help with defusion. Group members also frequently report an obsessive quality to their thoughts and compulsions such as repeating actions, counting, or rituals associated with these thoughts. Again, exploring this type of thinking in the group context can reduce isolation and reinforce the use of strategies such as exposure with response prevention. Group members will differ in their ability to notice their thoughts and beliefs, discuss their thoughts and experiences, and take alternative perspectives (cognitive flexibility). In this case, it is important to remind yourself that the therapeutic goal is not "correcting" thinking or completely getting rid of delusions (which is often not possible). The goals instead are to offer group members the experience of feeling heard and understood and the chance to enhance cognitive flexibility. Through the process of exploring and shifting thinking styles, group members improve their cognitive skills with the goal of personal growth and the ability to live a more value-consistent life.

The use of group process and group members' strengths-oriented and empowering feedback to one another is typically experienced as extremely beneficial and therapeutic. Individual postgroup follow-up to reinforce group learning and experiences is recommended. Given that group members progress at different rates, individual therapy for (some) clients postgroup can be a therapeutic option. Consistent with our approach and model, a compassionate, meaning-making, and empowering approach to working with distressing thoughts and delusions in a group context is the foundation for the group's process and progress.

Goals and Outline of Module (4 to 16 sessions)

As discussed, the therapeutic goals in working with distressing thoughts and delusions is to enhance value-consistent living and to work toward valued goals. By working through some of the barriers that distressing thoughts and delusions present clients can increase their ability to live a purposeful and meaningful life. By developing strategies to understand and address thoughts that get in the way of goal-directed behavior, clients can reduce the distress, time, avoidance, and limitation of activity associated with distressing thoughts and delusions. A reciprocal relationship can emerge where, through goal-directed activity, the impact of distressing thoughts and delusions can be minimized, and through less fusion, time, and preoccupation with distressing thoughts, goal-driven behavior can increase.

Overview of Treatment Area for Clinician

Psychoeducation around thinking and common thinking styles serves as a foundation for this module. We discuss the interconnected nature of thoughts, emotions, and behaviors, using an example depicted through the use of the CBT triangle. Discussion of the negative thinking bias in humans, which evolved to address threat or risk, can be extremely beneficial (see Hanson, 2013) as can the three emotional systems of threat, drive, and self-compassion/soothing (see Gilbert, 2009). We not only address the negativity bias but also positive psychology approaches of noticing and generating "positive" thoughts and emotions. We also offer a compassion-focused approach involving compassion-focused attention, thinking, and behavior exercises. See chapter 6 of this book, as well as Germer (2009), Gilbert (2009),

Gilbert & Choden (2013), Neff (2011), Tirch (2012), Welford (2012), and the books and websites in the "Positive Psychology" and "Compassion-Focused Therapy and Self-Compassion" sections in the Resources and on our website at http://www.treatingpsychosis.com.

As mentioned earlier, therapeutic work around distressing thoughts and delusions should proceed in a graded fashion, first addressing common thinking styles (see form 6.6) and then using a thought record or the 3/4Cs (form 6.7) to catch it (notice the thought), check it (explore alternative ways of thinking), and change it (shift thinking to what is more helpful or workable) with compassion. Through these exercises, common themes and distressing thoughts and delusions emerge. We use the terms "distressing thoughts" and "delusions" interchangeably to highlight the continuum conceptualization of thoughts and delusions as outlined below as well as to use language that "fits" best for clients.

What Are Delusions?

Delusions have been described as being false beliefs held in spite of evidence to the contrary and not in keeping with the individual's cultural, educational, or social background. They are described as not being amenable to reason (Sims, 1988). However, Kingdon and Turkington (1994) challenged the psychiatric community to reconsider the concept of delusion by questioning the veracity of each element of the definition. In 1996, Turkington, John, Siddle, Ward, and Birmingham developed a revised definition of delusion according to which *delusions* are beliefs that might be false but lie on the continuum of beliefs within society; may approximate to cultural, religious, or educational beliefs; and may show change in various parameters (for example, when explored within a collaborative setting). Delusions are split into secondary delusions and primary delusions. *Primary delusions* are typically functional in that they protect the sufferer from unbearable affect linked to schema vulnerability or undisclosed trauma. However, primary delusions can appear bizarre, are often systematized, and are characterized by delusional mood and delusional perception. We would echo Freud (1959) in agreeing about the rich meaningfulness of delusional content and would argue that on exploring the timeline (see the timeline exercise later in this chapter), we can understand the function and content of the delusion. We would therefore view the spectrum of human belief as being continuous but truncated at one end.

Secondary delusions are those that occur in response to some other phenomenon. They could be secondary to extreme sensitivity to stress leading to a hyperdopaminergic state, hallucinatory experiences, "unbearable" intrusive thoughts, déjà vu, depersonalization, or dissociation. The following are examples of secondary delusions:

In stress sensitivity: "Red cars on the road outside my house are keeping me under surveillance" or "Number plates with 6 in them are all meaningful to me personally."

In hallucinations: "The voices are those of aliens from a distant planet; they are going to torture me and then abduct me."

In intrusive thoughts of a sexual type: "A demon has possessed my mind and is making me think sexual thoughts."

In déjà vu: "I have the power of telepathy; I can transcend time."

In depersonalization: "My soul has been stolen by a coven of witches."

In dissociation: "A machine is switched on by the police and they make me disappear."

Although these are delusional beliefs, they are understandable, culturally syntonic explanations of real human experiences and biological shifts. Like primary delusions, secondary delusions such as these are excellent targets for intervention with the therapeutic approaches described in this chapter.

Not all delusions are bizarre. For example, delusional disorder can be characterized by nonbizarre delusions that are nevertheless extremely disabling. Examples may include thoughts like "I have the flu," "My nose is the wrong shape," or "My body emits a horrible odor"; and thoughts such as these may occur despite evidence to the contrary. These delusions can be more difficult to question and reality-test due to their cultural syntonicity. However, they can be worked with therapeutically—using a range of the therapeutic approaches described in this chapter to enhance social and other functioning—and contribute to work toward valued goals (Turkington et al., 1996).

Etiology of Delusions

Turkington and colleagues (2009) have argued that the human brain, from an evolutionary perspective, needs the production of new beliefs for society to advance in different situations and at different times. For example, the "delusion" of being in love results because love is crucial for mating to occur as well as to create a stable attachment base for the rearing of children. According to Turkington and colleagues, the capacity to develop delusions is therefore innately human. To survive as a species, flexibility is crucial. Therefore, we all have the capacity to experience delusions. It is not a mark of "insanity" but a crucial component of our humanity. There are biological propensities; delusions are more likely in those with a predisposing genetic vulnerability where sensitivity to stress mediates excessive dopamine production leading to delusion formation. Theory of mind deficits, attributional style, and a tendency to jump to conclusions can contribute (Bentall et al., 2009). Finally, cultural aspects are important. In China, delusions about courting and spitting are very common due to their unique cultural role, while these types of delusions are rarer elsewhere. An individual's schema formation is impacted by numerous factors, some of which are overt (for example, sexual abuse) and some of which are subtle (for example, misunderstandings by the child of environmental events). Triggering by key life events seems to be a pathway for some delusions.

Why Are Distressing Thoughts and Delusions Maintained?

Distressing thoughts and delusions can be maintained due to a number of reasons. It is important to identify and therapeutically target maintenance factors. This chapter (as well as others) addresses maintenance factors such as those listed below:

- Stress levels remain high, so dopamine levels remain elevated.

- Hallucinogens are repeatedly taken.

- The delusion is protecting against unprocessed affect.

- Safety behaviors have been activated due to distress caused by the individual's appraisals. Safety behaviors and avoidance strategies might include hypervigilance, social avoidance, self-harm, rituals, protective imagery (for example, a crucifix), thought suppression, and sleep deprivation.

- Dysfunctional coping strategies, such as listening to extremely loud and violent rap music or heavy metal, may have been activated.

- Individuals may receive positive reactions to their delusions from others that encourage the maintenance of the delusion. This can be particularly true of certain grandiose delusions—for example, a man believing that his mission was to destroy all the pornography in his hometown was strongly supported by local church groups.

- Individuals may generate negative reactions to their delusions from others that encourage the maintenance of the delusion. (For example, a woman who kept contacting her minister as she believed that he was in love with her was the subject of many negative statements by female parishioners. She took this as being definitive evidence that she was correct.)

Agenda for the Session

Check-In

Complete a check-in with your clients based on their functioning since the last session, including the day of the current session. The check-in can involve these ratings:

Mood rating 0–10 (10 being the highest level of positive mood)

Anxiety rating 0–10 (10 being the highest level of anxiety)

Self-efficacy or accomplishment rating 0–10 (10 being the highest level of self-efficacy)

Psychosis rating 0–10 (10 constituting the highest level of distress associated with thoughts or delusions and/or unusual experiences such as hallucinations—for example, voices).

Summary and Link to Previous Session

Summarize the material from the previous session on moving in the direction of valued goals by coping with the negative symptoms and defeatist beliefs that are often associated with limited goal-directed activity. In this module, it is important to emphasize distressing thoughts and delusions, including the defeatist beliefs addressed in the previous module and sessions. Link the between-session practice to the current session's topic. It can be helpful to notice any connection between negative symptoms and attempts to avoid distressing thoughts or delusions.

Review and Problem Solving of Between-Session Practice

Collaboratively review the between-session practice with your clients by reading through the session summary (form 5.1). Highlight accomplishments and progress made. In addition, problem-solve any difficulties that may have gotten in the way of starting or completing the practice.

Coping Exercise

Lead your clients in one of the coping exercises (see form 4.2). Give sufficient time to process the exercise and discuss any experienced benefits or drawbacks. Reinforce insights and positive or constructive elements of the experience.

Overview of Session/Topic Area for Clients

Provide a brief overview of the session content and rationale. Consistent with a normalizing approach, discuss the common nature of distressing thoughts and beliefs as well as thinking styles. Use language that speaks first to "distressing," "upsetting," or "unhelpful" thoughts. When clinically appropriate, discuss "delusions." Your clients may have heard this term but may not understand it fully. Discuss the definition from Turkington et al. (1996) that delusions are beliefs that might be false but lie on the continuum of beliefs within society. Also discuss the fact that delusions may approximate to cultural, religious, or educational beliefs and may show change in various parameters. Use the language that best fits your clients. If your clients do not agree with use of the term "delusions," you can replace that term with those above (or others that you collaboratively agree upon). Client-accepted language and respect for your clients' understanding and way of labeling their thoughts is essential.

Clinician Stance

A Collaborative Style for Working with Distressing Thoughts or Delusions

Your approach as clinician should be one of understanding, compassion, gentle questioning, conceptualization, and checking out thoughts. If appropriate, work on vulnerabilities to address the function of distressing thoughts and delusions (for example, the compensatory or self-esteem–enhancing function of delusions around specialness).

Engagement can be extremely difficult and depends on the degree of distrust, preoccupation, conviction, and emotional activation clients may be experiencing. It may not be possible to work in the classic CBT session structure of setting a goal, describing the CBT model, working on one target, generating a homework exercise, and then moving to a capsule summary and feedback. In the early sessions, your clients may well fill the session with upsetting material linked to the distressing thoughts or delusions. This needs to be handled with empathy and without attempting to press ahead with therapy goals too quickly. Compassion is crucial, as is a slow pace and avoiding being drawn into confrontation or collusion. In general, in the early sessions you "sit on the fence" in relation to the distressing thought or delusion. Often, homework will not be done. As clinician, you should ask if there is anything you might do or read to understand your clients' experience better. We can begin to set goals. However, your clients may set a goal related to the distressing thought or delusion (for example, "I want to stop the cult from sending me telepathy"). It might be possible to work on this by focusing on strategies to decrease activation and enhance distress tolerance.

Module Therapeutic Strategies and Exercises

This module provides several strategies and exercises for addressing distressing thoughts and delusions. Content and length of the module should be individualized for each client. The strategies discussed include the processes in our integrated theoretical model: values work, normalizing and accepting, present-moment awareness, self-as-context, defusion, cognitive reappraisal, mindfulness, compassion-focused approaches, and committed action. The therapeutic strategies discussed in this module are not exhaustive. Therapeutic approaches addressed in previous modules on emotion regulation and resilience and getting active can also be integrated in the work with distressing thoughts and delusions. Below we address a number of treatment approaches:

- Identification of goals and barriers to goal directed activity

- Understanding distressing thoughts, delusions, and delusional beliefs

- Normalizing distressing thoughts and delusions

- Conceptualization

- Metacognitive approaches

- Catching thoughts—a thought record, the 3 (or 4) Cs, and mindfulness

- Checking out and changing thoughts—alternative explanations and peripheral, inductive, and Socratic questioning styles, reality testing, and behavioral experiments

- Working at the level of core beliefs or schemas

- Compassion-focused approaches

Identification of Goals and Barriers to Goal-Directed Activity

Very often the generation of goals is not easy, as the distressing thoughts or delusions occupy so much of your clients' energy. Consider the following as examples of committed action toward goals:

- Getting out of the house

- Completing self-care activities even when feeling distressed by unusual thoughts, delusions, and/or voices

- Doing mindfulness or exposure exercises to reduce distress about thoughts or delusions in order to engage in goal-directed activity like exercise

- Engaging in compassion-focused exercises to reduce distress and increase ability to participate in a community group

- Going back to church or other faith group

Your clients' values can be used to help develop a rationale and motivation for committed action. Goal-directed activity is crucial for decreasing the impact of maintaining factors associated with psychosis, including avoidance, worry, rumination, and catastrophization. In addition, engagement in goal-directed activity enables clients to have experiences that are inconsistent with distressing thoughts and delusions. The early sessions therefore can be focused on activation through identifying values, working toward value-consistent living, and identifying and engaging in committed action toward valued goals.

Understanding Distressing Thoughts, Delusions, and Delusional Beliefs

—CLINICIAN EXERCISE————————

In the space below, write down the attitude you would have to the following client's beliefs:

> "The squidants are chimeras released by scientists. I heard on the radio that they are coming ashore and will kill the entire population. They will take over the government."

There is no right answer. This is, however, a high-conviction delusion causing extreme anxiety.

Useful Approaches

Curiosity: Could this be true or partly true?

Respect for the belief: We don't know everything that scientists are doing. Let's discuss it some more.

Empathy: I can see how distressed you are.

Risk consciousness: How can we make things feel safer for you while we check it out?

Guided discovery: I'm curious. Are you willing to check this out a bit more? How big are chimeras? Which bit of the squidant would be human and which bit squid? If the legs are human and the top a squid, that would be scary but its brain would be tiny. If the bottom half is squid and the top half human, then how could it move on dry land? (*Such an approach could lead to humor, but we need to be very careful with it.*)

Looking for triggers: What were you doing before you heard this on the radio? What channel were you on?

These styles are supportive and nonrejecting. They can take the heat out of the distressing thoughts or delusions and reduce threat.

Counterproductive Approaches

Collusion: "Yes, I own the factory, and we only released a few; they will be caught soon. The police are out shooting them now."

Confrontation: "You've been smoking weed again—you know this isn't possible. I may have to commit you to the hospital if this continues."

Humoring: "There, there now. Everything will be okay."

Ignoring: "What else is going on? Did you see the game last night? The New England Patriots won easily."

Working with Suspicious and Paranoid Thoughts

Move from abstract to concrete. Go from abstract terms to concrete ones. For example, "You say they're after you. Who is it that is after you?" It is important to extract as much detail as possible.

Reflect. Use plenty of reflection—that is, repeating back what you've heard. Not only does it help engagement by letting your clients know you've heard and understood what they said, but it also gives you time to think about how to proceed!

Gather evidence. What is the evidence for your clients' thoughts or beliefs? For example, "What makes you think that?"

Examine client conclusion. Is there anything that makes your clients think that they might have jumped to a conclusion or not considered different explanations?

Consider alternative explanations. Is there any other way of seeing things or of understanding the evidence? Consider alternative explanations. For example, "You say that you think that every time people touch their nose it's a code saying they think you're gay. Could there be any other explanation for why some people touch their noses?" If your client cannot come up with any alternative ways of seeing the situation, then you may need to provide a cue or generate alternatives. For example, "What would a friend or family member say?" "You have told me that there is a UFO hovering over your house every night. I know this might sound strange, but could it be a recurring vivid nightmare or a burglar light or some other local phenomenon?"

Use behavioral experiments. To test out both beliefs and alternative beliefs, use collaboratively generated behavioral experiments such as placing things in one's apartment in a certain way to see if anyone has entered the apartment.

Facilitate. Remember, your clients should do the thinking. This will be a process of guided discovery; you're just there to facilitate!

Understand the Experience of Psychosis

There are many things to keep in mind. Certain cognitive biases have been found to be associated with those who experience psychosis:

Jumping to conclusions. Clients with psychosis use less information before they make up their minds, so we are guiding them to consider other elements of evidence or alternative explanations.

Having an egocentric bias. For example, "The people on the bus are looking at me."

Having an intentionalizing bias. For example, "The neighbors want to get me."

Having an externalizing bias. For example, "People are after me" instead of "I feel scared."

It has been found that psychosis is associated with a tendency not to look for disconfirmatory evidence or information. This may be a resource-sparing strategy to cope with cognitive difficulties or deficits. In addition, it has been found that those with psychosis are less likely to have alternative explanations available to them without being guided to discover them.

Normalizing Distressing Thoughts and Delusions

Normalizing through psychoeducation can be very helpful for distressing thoughts and delusions, including secondary delusions and persecutory primary delusions. A client who reports that voices must come from God because they seem so powerful and knowledgeable can be empathized with. It is a reasonable conclusion in many cultures! Normalizing information about voices (for example, Turkington et al., 2009) will demonstrate how common voices are and how they can be managed with different coping approaches (Howard, Forsyth, Spencer, Young, & Turkington, 2013). Similarly, http://www .paranoidthoughts.com is a website that highlights that such beliefs are common and can change. Delusions of persecution can be linked to metabeliefs common in certain cultures that a paranoid mindset will keep you safe. Such metabeliefs can be demonstrated to be unnecessary in other cultural settings. For example, in some parts of Los Angeles being hyperalert to gang boundaries and expecting possible attack can be lifesaving, but is this true in Beverly Hills? It can therefore be very helpful to acknowledge that at one time in a client's life the paranoia was useful but may be less needed now. Here it can be useful to personally disclose if you have ever had a period of having an unusual belief that you have subsequently moved away from.

—CLINICIAN EXERCISE

Take a moment to think about a belief that you once held. Reflect on how you moved away from this belief. Here's an example from Dr. Turkington:

JFK cover-up: I will often tell patients that for a few years I was convinced that there was a massive cover-up around the JFK assassination. I found myself reading everything I could find and watching documentaries over and over again. Two things happened:

1. I realized that I was spending too much time thinking about it and would not find an answer.

2. New and compelling evidence that it was not a cover-up was published.

Now return to your own unusual belief. Please write below an example of an unusual belief that you once held and then explain how you moved away from this belief.

This approach is very useful in that clients see that the clinician is also "struggling" and is happy to disclose these ideas and how they shifted. Normalizing delusions shows that you, as clinician, are an open-minded person who won't make snap judgments. Normalizing also helps with negative metabeliefs about paranoia being linked to insanity and violence. We can all have unusual thoughts and negative metabeliefs. It is part of our common humanity.

Conceptualization

Conceptualization can be done using the ABC below and the approach outlined in chapter 5 with the conceptualization form (form 5.2). The use of a timeline as described in this chapter can be very informative and powerful. Highlighting strengths, coping strategies, and resources on form 4.3 should be an integral part of conceptualization and therapy work with distressing thoughts and delusions.

Clinical Example

A client, Eli, believes that his mother has been replaced by an identical replica. On a day-to-day basis, it can be conceptualized using an ABC:

Activating Event = (same in both examples)	Beliefs/Thoughts/Images About the Activity	Consequences (emotions and behaviors)
Distressing Belief:		
A person brings me my breakfast.	*She seems strange. She's an impostor.*	Emotions: *Feel angry* Behaviors: *Don't talk to her* *Avoid any contact*
Helpful Alternative/Belief:		
A person brings me my breakfast.	*She seems strange, but it doesn't seem likely she's an impostor. It must be my mom.*	Emotions: *Feel relieved* Behaviors: *Thank my mom*

With such a delusion, it is important to explore the meaning and function of the belief. An examination of the antecedents of the delusion showed that Eli's girlfriend told him that the child she was carrying wasn't his. This triggered the incresing anxiety he experienced upon returning to his mother's house, which led in turn to a delusional perception that she wasn't his real mother. Exploration of the timeline showed that his parents separated when he was eleven years of age. Eli never understood why he went to live with his father. He remembers feeling very abandoned by his mother. During inductive questioning, his clinician detected the thought that perhaps his real mother had been killed. With a full timeline, we can understand the functionality, meaning, and content of the delusion.

Metacognitive Approaches

Metacognitive approaches can be used to increase cognitive flexibility and perspective. *Metathinking*—that is, thinking about one's thinking—enhances cognitive flexibility through such processes as defusion, engaging in the stance of self as observer (an observer of one's thoughts), mindfulness and therapeutic strategies for the thinking styles of worry, rumination and self-criticism. We describe a number of metacognitive approaches below:

Mindfulness. This can be a very useful technique for coping with the stress of the delusion. As previously discussed, mindfulness can be taught by means of experiential exercises and practice in session. (For downloadable exercises, see our website http://www.treatingpsychosis.com.) Mindfulness should be clearly modeled by the therapist. Mindfulness is a skill to develop metacognitive awareness; it also functions as a form of exposure, as your clients are taught to sit with and nonjudgmentally observe their uncomfortable and distressing thoughts and feelings. This process reduces experiential avoidance and increases distress tolerance.

Worry or rumination postponement. Worry or rumination can be postponed until a "worry period." For example, clients are instructed to focus their attention and efforts on worry or rumination during a specified "worry time" or "rumination time." This time should be booked into their schedule for the day and should be time limited. For example, a fifteen- or thirty-minute worry period could be scheduled in for 6:00–6:15 p.m. or 6:00–6:30 p.m. each day. When thoughts arise about the delusion at other times of the day, worry about them is postponed until the designated period. This might allow time for some other goals to be achieved; it may also enhance perspective, defusion, and "reality testing."

Worry postponement with anxiety-causing delusions. With delusions that cause anxiety, worry postponement is strongly predicated by degree of conviction and level of insight. If insight is completely lost and conviction is 100 percent, then giving thirty minutes each day as prescribed worry time is unlikely to be successful. However, you can still discuss with your clients whether the worry is actually efficiently helping the situation.

Rumination postponement in relation to delusional systems. This tends to occur in relation to delusions that are seen as very meaningful. Tom, a World War II veteran who had served with the British Army in Egypt, had a delusional perception and came to believe that all of modern history was still being driven by a pharaoh somewhere in Egypt. He saw Egyptian symbols everywhere and spent his time ruminating on how the pharaoh was intervening to correct modern society. Perplexed and preoccupied, he had very little diversity in his life and experienced a low quality of life. Medication produced only minimal benefits. Obviously, if Tom could be helped to limit the time spent in rumination, other more meaningful goal-directed activities could be scheduled. Rumination postponement can be aided by imagery re-scripting, consideration of the key missing piece of evidence and what would happen if it were found, and mindfulness.

Criticism postponement in relation to critical hallucinations. Critical hallucinations very often echo critical self-talk and are schema syntonic—for example, "I am a failure and need repeated criticism"—making this a very problematic situation. The functions of criticism—whether the critical voice is acting to destroy or encourage the self—should first be explored. It is usually agreed that the voice is actually attempting to encourage. Hopefully, feeling less attacked, the client can establish a self-criticism time of fifteen minutes per day, so that the nature of the "encouragement" might be explored. This can be paralleled by schema therapy on the subject of failure using positive and negative logs, the continuum, and analysis of the evidence. A focus on gentle self-correction or constructive self-feedback, rather than self-criticism, can be emphasized.

Catching Thoughts: Thought Record, 3/4Cs, and Mindfulness

Catching or noticing thoughts or delusions is a very powerful strategy in beginning to shift client understanding of, and relationship and fusion with, distressing thoughts and delusions. This book presents a number of strategies for learning how to notice, catch, or track our thoughts. We have discussed the thought record and a simplified version of a thought record called the 3Cs in chapter 6. (Please see Greenberger and Padesky [1995] for the traditional thought record form.) We have found that the 3Cs (catch it, check it, change it) are a "catchy" and appealing way for clients (and ourselves!) to notice, or catch, distressing thoughts, delusions, and unhelpful thinking styles, and then start to check them out and change or shift them (see form 6.7). Mindfulness as described in chapter 6 can be used to notice and defuse from distressing thoughts. Mindfulness can involve taking more of a self-as-observer stance. Training in compassionate mind work and attention shifting can be conducted (see chapter 6 and the corresponding form 6.5 in the appendix). Returning to the breath in mindfulness can help enhance cognitive defusion as can attention training. (This could involve switching attention to the sound of a watch, traffic noise, the sound of the rain outside, and so forth.)

Checking Out and Changing Thoughts

Once clients have increased their ability to notice or catch thoughts, we can also begin therapeutic work on checking out thoughts through such approaches as considering alternative explanations, different questioning styles, reality testing, checking out the evidence, and behavioral experiments. As sessions proceed, you might ask your clients if there are any alternative explanations to their firmly held belief(s). One approach is to suggest the possibility of something unlikely, but close, in terms of content and bizarreness. If your client reports surveillance by Al-Qaeda, then you could ask, "If you're under surveillance, could it not possibly be by the Mafia, the CIA, or the tax authorities?" This is not collusion because it allows your clients to maintain their belief while considering other options, which can begin to be tested out in between-session practice. Your next question may query the types of cars these organizations might use if they had someone under surveillance. Through this approach you can begin to introduce doubt, which can then extend to further experiments relating to the issue of surveillance itself (see below). Peripheral, Socratic, and inference-based questioning styles can then be used to further introduce doubt. It is extremely useful to have a visual representation of these alternative explanations. The pie chart can be used as a helpful visual tool for collaboratively exploring alternative explanations (see form 8.2, Pie Chart for Alternative Explanations).

Conducting Behavioral Experiments

The use of behavioral experiments can be very helpful in exploring distressing thoughts and beliefs. Coming from a stance of curiosity and exploration, collaborative development of an "experiment" to test or check out thoughts and beliefs enhances the processes of developing cognitive flexibility and exploring the assumption that thoughts or delusions are facts. There are always at least two experiments. The first causes only mild anxiety (approximately a 20 percent increase) and is usually done at home. The second causes moderate anxiety (approximately a 40 percent increase) and normally is in the community. To assist you with behavioral experiments, please see form 8.3, Behavioral Experiments for Distressing Thoughts or Delusions, and keep these guidelines in mind:

- An effective coping strategy must have been learned beforehand.

- The client must be clear that the experiment can be stopped at any time and whatever has been learned can then be reviewed.

- Safety behaviors need to be suspended briefly in the hope of discovering more information.

Clinical Example

A client believed that there was a satellite removing his thoughts and broadcasting them to others. He was therefore too ashamed to leave his house except under cover of darkness.

Questions to explore alternative explanations:

- How often do you feel that your thoughts are removed and broadcast?

- How high can satellites go?

- What kind of orbits do they have?

- What are their functions? Can they broadcast thoughts?

- How long do they stay up for?

These questions are usually very interesting and not challenging for the client. It is often the case that the clinician won't know the answers, and the client and clinician will have to genuinely collaborate to discover them. Dr. Turkington describes below the approach he used with a client who had the belief being discussed—that a satellite was removing his thoughts and broadcasting them.

The first experiment we developed was to focus on the experience itself and give a fuller report. A simple diary of times and possible triggers helped us to see if there was any cyclical pattern that might fit with a satellite's orbit. It also helped us examine how powerful the experience was and led to conclusions of just how far the thoughts might reach. The experiment led the client to conclude that there was no cyclical pattern, so the satellite must have a stationary orbit over his house and that the broadcasting would be powerful enough to reach the local shopping center. Next, we decided to watch from his window and, when the thoughts were being broadcasted, he would think that President Obama had arrived and was doing a speech in the shopping mall. We concurred that if the thought were detected, we would see a definite measurable reaction of people being excited and all moving into the mall. It was important to outline what it would mean if they didn't react. Maybe not everyone could pick up the thoughts, maybe the range was less than we thought, or maybe the experience was a truly private one. All of these possibilities were encouraging because they might allow experimentation with more daytime social contact.

Working at the Level of Core Beliefs or Schemas

In the case example described earlier in which a man, Eli, believed his mother to have been replaced by a replica, work on the prepsychotic period revealed a trigger (his girlfriend indicated she was pregnant but not with his child) and a delusional perception (that his mother was not his real mother). Work on the timeline revealed a core belief or schema vulnerability linked to abandonment. This is the "hot schema," activated by the particular life event of being abandoned. If this event had not happened, the delusion would not have been needed at that point in time. The earliest description of this phenomenon was by Moorhead and Turkington (2001). The hot schema is protected by the delusion, and, as such, if we question too much or do too much schema-level work, a simple retreat into the delusion can be seen. This will slow progress. Guided discovery along with imagery work can be very helpful.

Guided Discovery

Clinician: You don't seem to have mentioned why your parents split up. Do you know anything about this or could we ask someone?

Client:	Well, I'm not asking the one at home!
Clinician:	Do you have grandparents or anyone else who might know something?
Client:	Now that you mention it, my aunt Jen was a regular visitor at our house and I could ask her.

Imagery Work

Clinician:	You have a very clear memory of being driven home to your father's from a meeting with your mother. Can we explore the memory further and see if you have any more details?
Client:	How can we do this?
Clinician:	Okay. I'll role-play your father. What was he wearing and what mood was he in? What kind of car was it? Was it a sunny day?
Client:	He had his denims on and wasn't talking. I remember now it was a dull day and all the leaves were falling off the trees. It was fall.
Clinician:	Where was your mother? When you met her, what was she wearing?
Client:	She was on her own, and my father wouldn't let me near her. We met at a cross-roads, and she was wearing different clothes. (*In tears*)

Here we are at the heart of the hot schema, and if the patient can tolerate the affect or return to it gradually, then the delusion becomes less necessary. We can then work on the emotional pain surrounding his girlfriend and the pregnancy. Note that usually such work cannot be done quickly and there will likely be episodic retreat into delusional safety.

Clinical Example

Consider the example of Mark, a twenty-four-year-old male who presented for therapy six months following his first psychotic experiences. He reported a delusion that his fiancée was having an affair with a local news anchorman and would leave him any day, although she indicated repeatedly that this was not the case. After exploring Mark's history, Mark and his clinician create the following timeline (see figure 8.1):

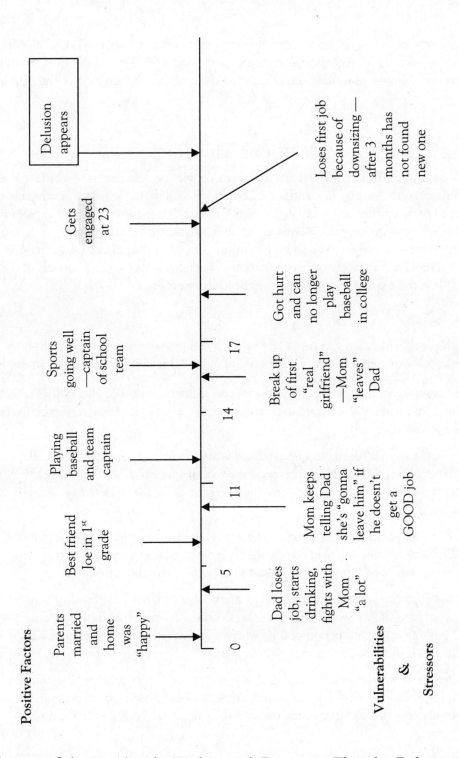

FIGURE 8.1   Timeline for Working with Distressing Thoughts/Delusions

Mark's timeline starts to demonstrate a vulnerability to possible abandonment in key relationships and also a compensatory striving for success in academics, sports, and work. With the help of the timeline, both Mark and the therapist now understand both the content and the function of the delusion better.

Distressing Thoughts or Delusions Timelines

The purpose of creating a timeline with clients with high-conviction delusions is to assist in developing the overall conceptualization and to identify core beliefs. (Recall that core beliefs or schemas are theorized to be formed between the ages of five and eleven.) This technique also allows for exploration of factors that may have influenced the development and maintenance of psychotic symptoms. Information gathered in the timeline may also be helpful in educating your clients about models of stress and coping and provides an excellent opportunity for normalizing. As with all aspects of CBT, this should be a collaborative exploration between the clinician and clients.

DIRECTIONS:

1. Explore with your clients what was going on in their lives approximately three months prior to the first psychotic experience. Identify emotions, automatic thoughts, stressors, and strengths.

2. Using inductive questioning, create age ranges for specific periods of your clients' lives. Again, collect further information about automatic thoughts, key emotions, stressors, protective factors, and achievements.

    •   Creating time periods based on school-related years can anchor your clients' recollections. For example, this might include ages zero to four (prior to school), five to eleven (elementary school), twelve to thirteen (middle school), and fourteen to seventeen (high school).

    •   For each age range, ask these questions: What was happening during that time of your life? What was it like at home? What were your key relationships? Note that it is important to access both positive and negative aspects of the client history.

    •   Ask about your clients' transition into elementary school: What was your first school like for you? How did you get along with others? Who were your friends in elementary school? Note that this is a period of time where children frequently experience bullying, which has been tied to negative outcomes later.

    •   Also keep in mind that middle school, developmentally, is a time when individuals may experience closer or romantic relationships. It's also a time when drug and/or alcohol use may start. Remember to continue to evaluate for both positive and negative experiences.

3. As you collect information for each time span and enter it on the timeline, write the positives (strengths) you and your clients identify on the top of the timeline in chronological order. Also

note the vulnerabilities for elementary school, middle school, and for high school under the line (using a different color for each time period). Finally, in the twelve months prior to the development of symptoms, record stressors identified. Do this in a third color, also under the line.

Compassion-Focused Approaches

Compassion-focused approaches are most effective when working with delusions associated with critical auditory hallucinations, which are in turn linked to shame and an underlying schema of self-blame. Such exercises are also pertinent in persecutory delusions where, in the face of constant perceived threat and hypervigilance, they promote self-soothing. They are viable in the face of the delusional system with a negative underlying core belief such as "I am a bad or unlovable person." Compassionate self-statements can be reinforced by compassionate imagery, compassionate letter writing to the self, or a compassion box containing items that nurture the self, such as key photographs, poems, music, and so on. (See chapter 6 for more compassion-focused strategies, as well as form 6.5.)

Between-Session Practice

As noted above, sessions in the negative symptoms and getting active module (see chapter 7) are structured with the problem solving, processing, and planning of between-session practice as an explicit focus. Your between-session practice plan for the week will flow naturally from this discussion.

Feedback from Client on the Session

Ask your clients for constructive feedback on the session, including how it felt to talk about distressing thoughts or delusions. Address affect that may have been activated by discussion of these thoughts and beliefs, and honor the meaning and role these have played in your clients' experience of self and others. Finish sessions with feedback to the client about the courage and strength it takes to share these thoughts and experiences. As always, reinforce your clients' strengths, efforts in session, and movement toward their values and goals.

Summary of Session

Summarize the session for your clients and provide them with a written copy of this material (see form 5.1). Be sure to reinforce your clients' openness to challenges, their efforts, strengths, and accomplishments in writing, both on the session summary form (5.1) and the strengths form (4.3).

Ask your clients to read over the session handout at home and share this handout with family, friends, or caregivers. Model a strengths-focused approach by asking clients to identify one personal strength, quality, or accomplishment from the session. If your clients find it difficult to do so, you can cue with examples you have noticed or ask what a friend or family member might say. This reinforces your clients' efforts, strengths, accomplishments, and progress, and introduces the coping or grounding exercise.

Coping Exercise (Optional)

See form 4.2 in the appendix for examples.

Additional Resources

For more information, please see the Resources section of this book. You will find many of the forms in the appendix; they are also available for download at http://www.newharbinger.com/24076. (See the back of this book for instructions on how to access them.) Additional materials not available in this book can be found on our website at http://www.treatingpsychosis.com.

CHAPTER 9

Module 6: Understanding and Working with Voices

In this module, we highlight the therapeutic exploration and understanding of the experience of hearing voices. For clarity's sake, we have divided the chapter into two parts: part 1 deals with understanding and assessing voices, while part 2 addresses working with voices in therapy. A thorough understanding of the voice-hearing experience is critical to the work we do with both voices and other hallucinations. Voices often distract from valued life goals by consuming our clients' emotional energy and time. Through exploration, we gently engage in a connecting and validating form of exposure. Through this exploration, both you and your clients gain greater insight into your clients' understanding and experience of their voices. This understanding is then used to address barriers to working toward valued goals and impacts on the client beliefs about self, others, and the future. We start with an experiential exercise to enhance understanding of the lived experience of hearing voices and follow with a monitoring strategy for voices, the Voice Diary (form 9.1). The chapter then addresses relevant assessment questions. The value-informed compassionate approach to understanding and assessing voices lays the foundation for the therapeutic work with voices, which is covered in the second part of this chapter.

Materials

See appendix for forms. They are also available for download at http://www.newharbinger.com/24076. (See the back of this book for instructions on how to access them.) Because the cognitive abilities and needs of clients vary, we've provided additional versions of some forms in this chapter on the New Harbinger website.

Modifications for Group Implementation

Group approaches to working with voices can be conceptualized in a similar manner to working with distressing thoughts and delusions. Given the shame and self-stigma often associated with voice hearing, psychoeducation about the common nature of voice hearing in the general population as well as sharing in group about voices can be extremely depathologizing. Clients often report that the sense of not being alone in their experience of voices and the feeling of a common humanity with other clients are some of the most powerful and healing parts of the group. As with other topics or areas, clients share their experience at a pace that they determine. Some clients may be extremely hesitant and fearful about sharing the content of their voices particularly if they are of a violent or sexual nature. Psychoeducation around the common nature of intrusive violent or sexual thoughts is extremely helpful in addressing concerns or fears regarding the content of voices. A normalizing approach to the common human experience of intrusive thoughts is both reassuring and informative. Clients benefit from an emphasis on the idea that the content of voices (or intrusive thoughts) in and of itself does not mean that the client does or must agree with them. Such content is distressing due to the intrusive and egodystonic nature of the experience of violent or sexual thoughts or voices. A compassionate, normalizing, and empowering approach to working with voices in a group context is inherently therapeutic.

PART 1: Understanding Voices

—EXPERIENTIAL EXERCISE FOR VOICES—

For those clinicians who wish to have a better understanding of the experience of voices, the experiential exercise below can foster great insight. Although it may seem apparent how voices might affect someone's attention, concentration, engagement, and experience of self, this exercise can be a powerful tool to enhance understanding and empathy.

Ask colleagues or a couple of friends to try this exercise with you. Each person takes a turn being the voice, the voice hearer, and the clinician. The person who plays the role of the voice talks incessantly into the voice hearer's ear, repeating denigrating and/or hurtful statements, and/or making threats. The clinician engages in discussion with the voice hearer, asking questions and generally trying to engage. Usually a few minutes can give the person in the voice hearer role a sense of the struggle to focus and engage, the threatening and demoralizing experience of repeated negative statements, and the confusion and distress around threats. Ensure that by the end of this exercise each person has had the experience of each of the three roles. Debriefing together is essential to discuss the emotional and functional experience of being in the voice hearer and other roles.

Exploration and Assessment of Voices

Exploration of clients' experience of voices is a gentle process, guided by the clients' particular pace and sense of safety while building on previous therapeutic work with distressing thoughts. Delicate questioning and exploration through the use of the Voice Diary are important to initiate the exploration process for voices. The use of assessment measures, including symptom measures, to guide clinical exploration and evaluation can be very informative and clinically useful. Assessment measures can be used to begin exploration of voices, the themes of voices, and the clients' experience. In addition, assessment measures can be used to explore voices and beliefs about voices that are difficult for the client to access or discuss.

Assessment Areas and Questions

Areas to cover in the assessment of voices are listed below. (See also Coleman & Smith, 2005, and form 4.1.) Wording, pacing, and tone are important. The order and number of questions explored collaboratively by you and your clients is based on clinical judgment and client input around pacing. Some clients and clinicians find it more helpful to start with the Voice Diary, while others find exploration, normalization, and understanding through clinician questions helps their clients be more open and able to complete the Voice Diary work.

- **Understanding of voices:** your clients' explanation for, understanding of, and/or beliefs about the cause of the voices, why they hear voices, the voices' origins, and so on

- **Dimensions of voices:** frequency, loudness, conviction, pervasiveness, and so on

- **Characteristics of voices:** location, gender, vision with voices, distinctness versus mumbling, whether they come from self or are external to self, whether it's your client's own voice or another person's voice, whether voices heard through ears or elsewhere, the ability of others to hear the voices

- **Quality of voices:** punishing, encouraging, negative, positive, neutral, or other qualities

- **Pattern to voices:** predisposing factors, precipitators, perpetuators, situations, and so on

- **History of voices:** when the voice started vs. voice has always been there, precipitators or stressors preceding first voice hearing experience (cuing with stressors—use of drugs, trauma, loss, school/work problems, physical illness, and so on) can be important

- **Current voices:** voice profile for each voice

- **Content of voices:** wording of the voices and themes of what the voices say

- **Beliefs about voices:** content, cause, pros and cons of focusing on voices, power, control, and so on

- **Command voices:** risk, ways of responding, power differential, omnipotence, and so on

- **Relationship with voices:** antagonistic, demeaning, threatening-submissive, mutually threatening, persecutory-submissive, mutually friendly or caring

- **Altered consciousness with voices:** loss of time, flashbacks, and so on

Of note, not all of the assessment areas listed need to be covered at the outset of therapy or during the therapy process. Other areas of assessment may also be informative. Individualization and pacing are essential. As always, respect for your client's experience, including concerns and fears about talking about the voices, is critical. Respect your clients' verbal and nonverbal indications around pacing. The above information about voices can be collected through discussion and/or through using the Voice Diary (form 9.1).

The Voice Diary

The Voice Diary is a key assessment tool that can be used to understand and explore voices (see form 9.1). The experience of noticing and recording voices is important, as it enhances perspective and understanding and is a form of gentle exposure to voices. Understandably, clients frequently engage in experiential avoidance of voices. Your clients may try to avoid situations, events, or thoughts and feelings associated with voices in an attempt to "control" them and the associated experiences of distress. (Please refer to part 2 of chapter 9 for greater detail about mindfulness and acceptance-based approaches used with voices.) Completion of the Voice Diary can increase understanding and insight around the voice hearing experience. The exercise of completing the Voice Diary can be empowering in and of itself. Completing it can provide your client with some distance and objectivity. Completion of the Voice Diary can be a part of the voice exposure process and implicitly involves decreasing forms of experiential avoidance. Clients may have limited their lives to a great degree to try to avoid hearing distressing voices. Similar to individuals with phobias or fears, avoidance can work in the short term but actually increases fears, limits activities, and can be extremely disempowering.

Selected Assessment Measures for Voices

Engagement, assessment, and treatment all involve exploring—in a respectful, compassionate, and thorough way—the multiple dimensions of voices with a particular focus on beliefs about voices. The Beliefs About Voices Questionnaire–Revised (BAVQ–R; Chadwick, Lees, & Birchwood, 2000) is a useful clinical tool. It can be used to identify beliefs about voices that are disempowering or distressing, and can be used to assess changes in beliefs about voices over the course of therapy. The Psychotic Symptom Rating Scales (Haddock, McCarron, Tarrier, & Faragher, 1999) is a clinical and evaluation tool to look at the various dimensions of voices (and delusions). The Structured Clinical Interview for the Positive and Negative Syndrome Scale (SCI-PANSS) by Opler, Kay, Lindenmayer, & Fiszbein (1992) is a useful broader-based tool for assessing positive and negative symptoms. A section of the SCI-PANSS focuses specifically on "hallucinatory" behavior and associated delusions; it is not, however, as specific around the various dimensions of hallucinations as the Psychotic Symptom Rating Scales. For those who hear voices, struggle with command hallucinations, or have a power issue with their voices, the Voice Power Differential Scale (Birchwood, Meaden, Trower, Gilbert, & Plaistow, 2000) and the Risk of Acting on Commands Scale (Trower, Birchwood, Meaden, Byrne, Nelson, & Ross, 2004) can be valuable clinically. The Dissociative Experiences Scale (Bernstein & Putnam, 1986) helps to determine if there is a change in consciousness associated with the voices. For further information about clinical/evaluation measures, see our companion website at http://www.treatingpsychosis.com.

Part 2 of this chapter focuses on working with the perceived power of voices and understanding and dealing with command hallucinations. The Young Schema Questionnaire (Young & Brown, 1994) is extremely useful to get a better understanding of schemas or core beliefs that may drive the content and understanding of your clients' voices and your clients' relationship with their voices. The Young Schema Questionnaire can also be helpful in exploring the role of schema or core belief compensation and experiential avoidance. The downward arrow technique can also be used to uncover underlying core beliefs or schemas. Briefly, the downward arrow involves asking question after question about what it would mean about the self (the client) if certain automatic thoughts were true. Through this approach, one is typically able to get closer and closer to the underlying core beliefs or schemas that may drive voices, voice content, and the clients' responses to their voices.

To begin the downward-arrow technique, the clinician could say to their client, "I'm curious. Would you be willing to explore what your voices say a little bit more?" The following exchange gives an example of the downward- arrow technique:

Client: "My voices are incredibly critical of me."

Clinician: "I understand it might be hard, but would you be willing to tell me a bit more about what the voices actually say?"

Client: "Sure. The voices say I always do things wrong."

Clinician: "What do you think about what they say?"

Client: "I think it's true."

Clinician: "What would it mean if you always did things wrong?"

Client: "That I always screw things up."

Clinician: "And if that were true, what would it mean about you?"

Client: "That I'm a loser."

Clinician: "And if you were a loser, what would that mean?"

Client: "That I'm a complete failure, and I'll never be good enough for anyone."

By asking questions using the downward arrow technique, core beliefs or schemas are identified. These beliefs and the associated feelings can then be addressed therapeutically.

Areas to cover in a clinical assessment were addressed in chapter 4. As with other distressing experiences or symptoms, it is important to explore predisposing, precipitating, and perpetuating events associated with voices. As with the assessment of delusions, gentle exploration of client history and any stressors or triggers leading up to the first experience of voices is important. The history typically gives a context for the clients' experience and is very helpful in understanding the content and themes of the voices, the clients' understanding of the voices, and their response to, and relationship with, the voices. As Coleman and Smith (2005) indicate, stimulating a curiosity about the voices can lead to a decrease in distress and discomfort about the voices, can enhance ownership, and can reduce self- and other-stigma around voices. By creating an environment of safe exploration, your clients' understanding of their voice hearing experience can be enhanced. Understanding of the voices can be enhanced by discussing your clients' previous experiences, stressors or life problems, and personal traumas. (Stabilization and pacing are critical. See the paper on trauma on our companion website at http://www.treatingpsychosis.com.)

When discussing or exploring voices it is, of course, important to come from a shared stance that the voice experience is real for your clients. The purpose of the exploration and work with voices is an enhanced understanding of your clients' experience and explanation for their voices. This understanding can lead to greater acceptance of the voice hearing experience and a greater ability to cope with voices that allows clients to live more meaningful and goal-directed lives. If your clients experience less distress associated with (previously) disturbing voices and/or a different relationship with their voices, the content and beliefs about voices often shift, and the frequency, loudness, conviction, and intrusiveness of the voices often decreases.

Case Example: Jed

Jed, a single university student in his early twenties, was referred for therapy by student health services, as he was having a hard time concentrating on his studies and was feeling down and hopeless. Jed also reported concerns regarding contamination and the need to wash repeatedly, in which he was encouraged by voices that denigrated him.

Jed entered therapy somewhat reluctantly. However, over the course of many months, Jed began to share more in therapy. He reported feeling safer and more heard and understood with his current therapist than he had with other health care providers. Jed gradually began to share his history of sexual abuse and denigration, including his abuser soiling him as a child. Through gentle exploration within the safety, respect, and understanding of the therapeutic relationship, Jed was gradually able to make a connection between his history of abuse and his core belief of being bad, dirty, and contaminated. Jed was also able to connect his experience of denigrating voices with his core belief of being bad and dirty, which he linked to his history of abuse. Through therapy, Jed was better able to "make sense" of his compulsion to wash repeatedly, given his history of being soiled and his associated core belief around contamination. Jed described the experience of making links among his history, beliefs, and voice experiences as profoundly depathologizing. He said he could finally make sense of the voices, the content of which he had not previously shared with anyone. Jed indicated that, as a result of making these links, he felt less alone, had less shame, and had a greater understanding of himself and his voices. Jed indicated that he no longer felt as threatened by his voices and had developed a greater understanding, and acceptance, of his voice hearing experience. As a result of these insights in therapy, Jed was more able to engage in therapeutic exposure work on his compulsion to engage in washing rituals.

This kind of collaborative linking of voices to past history can be very powerful and normalizing for the client. Clients will often experience a kind of "eureka" moment in which they no longer judge the content of their voices as "crazy" but more as an understandable response to their past. Greater understanding and perspective can then open up the possibility of looking at the credibility of the voice content and can reduce self-stigma and enhance self-compassion around voice hearing.

Conceptualization of Voices Within the Integrated Treatment Model

The conceptualization flows out of the engagement and assessment process and can be integrated into the psychoeducation around the integrated treatment approach for voices (see chapters 2, 4, and 5). The conceptualization serves multiple purposes. It helps to establish an understanding of your clients' history and the evolution of core beliefs that may fuel the content of the voices. The act of collaboratively developing the conceptualization can be very empowering and depathologizing for your clients. When clients make a connection between their voices and past experience, the voice experience can make more sense to your clients (as well as family or caregivers). Thus, the conceptualization can help make sense of what can be seen as "non-sense." Through the conceptualization process, the voice can be seen as an understandable response to your clients' past rather than something irrational and "crazy." Through a greater understanding of why voices say what they do, clients experience compassion and empathy from you (and, through compassionate mind training, for themselves). In addition, the conceptualization process typically enhances engagement and your clients' openness to exploring and working with their voices. Frequently, when clinicians (and clients) get off track or are unsure of where to go in therapy, returning to the conceptualization can provide direction for the treatment trajectory.

Finally, the conceptualization process not only enhances your and your clients' understanding of the meaning and relevance of the voice content and how it might be linked to your clients' past, but it also provides insight into how voices are linked to your clients' values and goals. Conceptualization is a dynamic process that serves as the map or compass for the treatment. The conceptualization process evolves through greater client and clinician understanding as well as progression in therapy.

The components of the ACT part of our integrated conceptualization are adapted from Hayes, Strosahl, and Wilson (2012) and Harris (2009). Clarifying questions link your clients' previously identified valued directions with the barriers to valued living associated with the voices. For example, barriers in three areas for voices are listed below:

1. Fusion with voice content or fusion with beliefs about the origin of voices

2. Avoidance of voices or goal-directed activities due to a focus on voices

3. Unworkable action, such as arguing with the voices

The cognitive behavioral component of the conceptualization for voices outlined below is based on Judith Beck's (1995; 2011) theoretical framework and was modified for work with voices. See chapter 5 for an explanation of how to develop and use the integrated conceptualization to drive treatment planning.

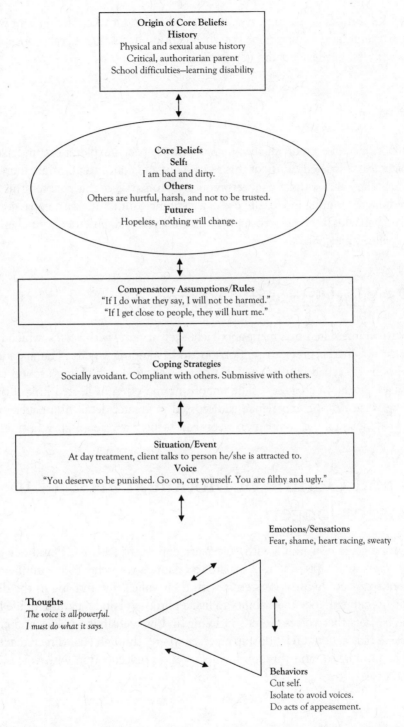

FIGURE 9.1   Sample Cognitive Behavioral Conceptualization for Voices. (Modified from Beck, 1995.)

Figure 9.1 illustrates an example of a conceptualization for voices for a client who had experienced a history of trauma and denigration. For therapeutic purposes, a blank conceptualization form for voices can be found in the appendix (form 9.2).

Summary

The importance of an individualized, appropriately paced exploration, understanding, and assessment of voices was discussed. Without this assessment and conceptualization, foundational therapeutic work can be limited and at times counterproductive. In part 2 of this chapter, this exploration of voice hearing provides the foundation for the use of acceptance, mindfulness, compassion-focused, and other cognitive and behavioral therapeutic approaches with voices to enhance your clients' movement in the direction of valued life goals.

Part 2: Working with Voices

We now focus on integrated treatment approaches for working with voices, which build directly on the content discussed in the previous section on understanding voices. Therapeutic work with voices should always be preceded by psychoeducation as well as skill building around coping and emotion regulation as discussed in chapter 6. The important and often neglected link of trauma and dissociation with the voice hearing experience is discussed in greater detail in a paper we have provided on trauma and psychosis on the companion website at http://www.treatingpsychosis.com.

Goals and Outline of Module, Part 2 (4 to 12 sessions, or longer)

The therapeutic goals in working with voices are consistent with ACT and our integrated model as described in previous chapters. The goals are to enhance your clients' meaning and sense of purpose through identifying and living consistently with their values and moving in the direction of a valued life. Your clients can enhance their ability to live a purposeful and meaningful life by working through some of the barriers that voices present in living and by identifying values and committed action to valued goals. A bidirectional relationship emerges where, through goal-directed activity, the impact of voices can be minimized, and through less focus and preoccupation with voices, valued goal-driven behavior increases.

Agenda for the Session(s)

Discuss the agenda for the session with your client. Collaboratively decide on the amount of content and number of skills to be covered in the session, factoring in time for check-in and any issues, especially those of a more urgent nature, that may have arisen between sessions. Also include a review and problem solving of between-session practice. Any issues that have come up can be placed on the agenda and linked to the session topic and content. Pacing is essential. Checking in with your client for feedback during the session and at the end of the session facilitates appropriate pacing of the sessions and material covered. Pacing and individualization often address overstimulation; however, checking in for feedback can also provide the opportunity for clients to give input when pacing is too slow or not engaging. To facilitate collaboration, ask your clients in each session whether there is anything they would like to put on the agenda.

Check-In

Complete a check-in with your clients based on their functioning since the last session, including the day of the current session. The check-in can involve the following ratings:

Mood rating 0–10 (10 being the highest level of positive mood)

Anxiety rating 0–10 (10 being the highest level of anxiety)

Self-efficacy or accomplishment rating 0–10 (10 being the highest level of self-efficacy)

Psychosis rating 0–10 (10 constituting the highest level of distress associated with thoughts, delusions, and/or hallucinations such as voices).

Ratings can also be added for belief in cause, content, and power of voices; control related to the voices; worry about, rumination about, or avoidance of voices; as well as time spent focused on voices rather than on valued goals.

Summary and Link to Previous Session

Summarize the material from the previous session and link it to the between-session practice and this session's topic. The link between distressing thoughts and voices is an extremely important one. Distressing thoughts or delusional beliefs about voices can increase distress. This link is highlighted later in this module to emphasize that it is not the voices themselves that cause distress but the thoughts or beliefs about the voices that impact on emotions and unhelpful behavior.

Review and Problem Solving of Between-Session Practice

Collaboratively review the between-session practice with your client. Also collaboratively problem-solve any of the barriers or difficulties raised. Continue to reinforce the importance of between-session or "real-life" practice. An analogy such as taking soccer lessons but not partcipating in a game between soccer lessons is a good example. (Try to modify examples to your clients' interests, such as playing a musical instrument or learning a particular new sport.)

Coping Exercise

Lead your client in one of the coping/grounding exercises (see form 4.2). Given the association between voices and a history of trauma, be aware of any potential issues for clients with a history of trauma.

Overview of Session/Topic Area for Clients

Provide a brief overview of the session content and rationale. The content should be targeted at the appropriate level for your client and the amount of content tailored for your client. Individualization is key!

Clinician Stance

Your stance should be one of understanding, compassion, and encouragement. Given that it can be extremely scary to talk about voices and that many clients' experience of voices has been invalidated, pacing needs to be within a therapeutic window that is not too activating. Clinicians should be aware of the potential that clients' voices will comment on them, or that command voices will tell clients not to talk about voices in therapy or go to therapy at all. Express caring and empathy around the courage it can take to talk about voices. Provide copious support around the process of sharing about voices, and ensure that feedback from clients throughout the process of working with voices is encouraged and requested.

Therapeutic Strategies and Exercises

The therapeutic strategies for voices are completed with the client in a manner consistent with the integrated model—that is, voices (or other hallucinations) are addressed as part of the overarching therapeutic purpose of working toward valued goals. Voices are addressed if they act as a barrier to living a value-consistent life and/or achieving goals, or if they impinge on quality of life due to the level of distress associated with them. Instead of working directly with the voices (for example, exploring their identity, content, relationship), you can focus therapeutic work on the core beliefs that drive the theme and content of the voices (such as those underlying low self-esteem or self-worth) and address these core beliefs first (or exclusively). It is critical to understand what purpose the voices may serve for your clients. By constructively addressing the purpose of the voices and developing skills and strategies to meet this need, we address the compensatory function the voices may have. For example, if the voices serve as company for your client, therapeutic work on enhancing social skills and social interaction can be conducted to diminish the need for the voice to serve this role. A focus on valued goals can redirect energies from preoccupation with voices to more meaningful pursuits. Exploring the advantages and disadvantages of the amount of time and energy spent on voices can help your clients to engage in more meaningful goal-directed activity or committed action. Of particular note, it is frequently necessary to address fears about risk associated with the voices before more acceptance- and mindfulness-based approaches can be implemented. Therefore, in this chapter we work with motivation (through values work), fear, control and power related to voices (through such strategies as examining the evidence, behavioral experiments, and exposure), and then move into more acceptance-, mindfulness-, and compassion-focused approaches. All of these exercises and approaches involve reducing avoidance, which enhances cognitive flexibility and reduces fusion.

Clients will often believe the external nature of the voice and the content due to a number of factors such as the "realness" of the voice. For example, your clients may report that the voice "sounds exactly like a family member," "says things that no one else could know," "knows things that I don't know," "is extremely detailed," and so on. Drawing a parallel with dreams or nightmares can be helpful for perspective taking—that is, voices sound real and authentic in dreams, and sometimes dreams have detail and information that the dreamer was not aware of. Just because the voice sounds real, does that make it truly an external voice? Does this mean the content is accurate or true? You can validate the "realness" of the person's experience while still leaving room to explore the cause, origin, content, and so on.

Psychoeducation About Voices

Consistent with the cognitive behavioral approach, psychoeducation about voices and the integrated treatment model is critical. Psychoeducation about voices can be an extremely normalizing, depathologizing, and destigmatizing process. Inform your clients about how common voices are, including the percentage of people who experience voices—that is, 4 to 25 percent of the general population and 71 percent of university students (see Beck et al., 2009)—and how common the voice experience is under certain conditions such as sleep deprivation, grief, trauma, and so on. Examples—such as that people put in a sensory deprivation tank for a long enough number of hours will begin to hallucinate—can be helpful for normalization purposes. A discussion of hypnagogic and hypnopompic hallucinations (that is, dream mentation experienced upon sleep onset or awakening, respectively) can also be very normalizing.

Next, educate your clients about the conceptualization of ideas or delusions on a continuum and indicate that the same understanding can be applied to how we experience beliefs about voices. Information mentioned above that your clients think may be a helpful reminder can be recorded by them on a coping card (with assistance by you in session; see the section on coping cards later in this chapter). As described in part 1 (on the understanding of voices), the psychoeducation and conceptualization process helps clarify the potential causes or precursors to voice hearing and beliefs about voices.

In addition, it can be helpful to educate your clients about cognitive distortions that can be more common in people who have a diagnosis of schizophrenia or have psychotic experiences. Beck et al. (2009), in their summary of the research, indicate that people with psychoses have the tendency to jump to conclusions with less information and less consideration, particularly during times of stress. In addition, research indicates that people who experience psychoses have more difficulty monitoring or identifying the source of noises. People who experience psychoses have also been found to have an *externalizing bias* (a tendency to attribute causes externally), a *personalizing bias* (a tendency to believe experiences and acts are related to self), and an *intentionalizing bias* (a tendency to attribute negative intentions to others). Discuss this information judiciously, with links to the implications for your clients. These cognitive distortions speak to the critical role of developing perspective-taking skills and greater flexibility in thinking with those who experience psychoses. The following sections speak to some of the perspective-taking and critical-thinking strategies (defusion strategies) that can be implemented collaboratively with clients around the understanding, cause, and credibility of the voices.

The ABC Model of Voices

In our integrative model, we work on enhancing cognitive flexibility through the use of diffusion strategies as well as directly looking at other possible explanations or understandings of the voice hearing experience. Completion of the ABC Model of Voices (fig. 9.2 below) and the ABC Voices form (9.3) helps your clients come to a greater understanding that it is not the voice itself that causes (a) the distress and (b) the behavioral response; it is the belief *about* the voice. Initiating therapeutic voice work around the role of beliefs about voices can enhance motivation and engagement. Further exploration of voices can engender a sense of hope and empowerment around how your clients understand and respond to their voices. Using the ABC model and a number of the exposure exercises can lay the foundation for the more acceptance-oriented therapeutic work.

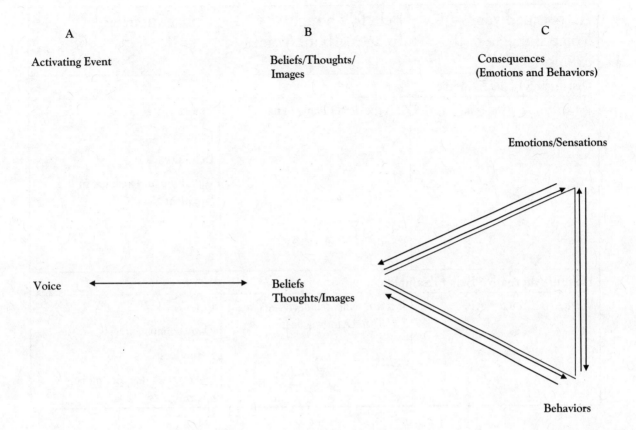

A	B	C
Activating Event	Beliefs/Thoughts/Images	Consequences (Emotions and Behaviors)

FIGURE 9.2   ABC Model of Voices

An absolutely critical piece for understanding the ABC Model of Voices is that the voice itself is the activating event. It is the beliefs, thoughts, and/or images about the voice that determine the emotional (feeling) and behavioral consequences. As shown in figure 9.2, feelings, behaviors, and beliefs or thoughts are all interrelated—that is, there is a "multidirectional" relationship among beliefs, feelings, and behaviors that can develop into a feedback loop that is self-reinforcing. Enhance understanding of the model by using an example generated by your clients. For example, clients who report a voice that says "you are evil" can look at their thoughts, beliefs, and/or images about the content of the voice and how their thoughts, beliefs, and/or images impact on how they feel (fearful) and behave (withdrawing and lock self in basement). Drawing the ABC model on a whiteboard should be done as a collaborative process. The use of a client example for completing the ABC Voices form (9.3) in session can be very powerful and informative.

Activating Event = Voice (same in both examples)	Beliefs/Thoughts/ Images About Voices	Consequences
Distressing Belief Example:		
Voice says, "You are evil."	*It is the devil talking to me.*	Emotions: *Fear, shame* Behaviors: *Withdraw and lock self in basement*
Helpful/Alternative Belief Example:		
Voice says, "You are evil."	*It is not really the devil speaking. I don't have to believe it.*	Emotions: *Okay, competent* Behaviors: *Get on with day and move toward goals*

FORM 9.3 ABC FOR VOICES FORM: EXAMPLE

Clients are asked to recall a voice they heard in the recent past. The exact wording of this voice is written down in both row A (the distressing belief example) and row B (the balanced or alternative belief example). In both cases, the activating event (the voice) is exactly the same. In this example, the voice says, "You are evil." Ask your clients what their usual (distressing) belief about the content of the voice is, and then ask them to consider the typical emotional and behavioral consequences associated with this belief. Following this, you can ask your clients to generate an alternative or more balanced belief about the content of the voice that says, "You are evil." If your clients have difficulty generating another belief, you can help by using various perspective-taking techniques.

- What belief might a friend, family member, or health care professional hold about this voice?

- What have others said in the past about what the voice says?

If your clients are unable to come up with an alternative belief, you can offer a number of potential thoughts or beliefs. Then ask your clients what the consequences would be, from a feeling and behavioral perspective, if this "alternative" belief were true. Once the exercise is complete and the form filled in, you can explore the outcome Socratically with your client. The following types of questions can be used:

- What do you make of this exercise?

- What do you notice about the emotional and behavioral consequences in each example?

- What made a difference in how you felt and behaved?

Therapeutic Approaches
Working with Beliefs About Voices

After completing the ABC Model of Voices together, you can then engage your client in completing the ABC for Voices form (form 9.3). Filling out the ABC for Voices form (9.3) with your clients sitting by your side enhances the collaborative coexploration stance of the therapy with the goal of enhancing cognitive flexibility around voices and decreasing fusion. Filling out the form can help with understanding and consolidation as your clients can take the completed form home and refer back to their ABC Model of Voices.

Reinforcement and repetition is critical in therapy. Given the cognitive biases described above, it is important to give your clients repeated opportunities to explore their beliefs about the content of the voices as well as repeated opportunities to explore and consider other possible understandings or explanations.

Another perspective-taking and distancing exercise is to collaboratively explore with your clients the advantages and disadvantages to their current beliefs about voice content (see form 9.4, Pros and Cons of Beliefs About the Content of Voices). By "taking a step back," your clients are able to become more objective about or defuse from their thinking—that is, your clients are able to think about their thinking. Metacognitive approaches such as these can be very helpful in providing greater insight.

Collaborative Socratic exploration of evidence for and against beliefs about voices can be done through the use of the Evidence for and Against Beliefs About the Content of Voices form (9.5). The process of looking for evidence for and against beliefs can be very informative for clients and can give them yet another experience of perspective taking or defusion. When completing form 9.5 with your client in session, it is advisable to start with evidence for your clients' beliefs. By doing so, you enhance engagement and demonstrate a respect for, and openness to, their experience and thoughts.

Following completion of the ABC for Voices form and the other exercises and forms above (which focus on the beliefs and thoughts about the content of the voices), you can complete another form exploring your clients' beliefs or thoughts about the origin or cause of the voices (form 9.6). The same procedure can be used as was used with the beliefs about voice content—that is, completing the form in session together first and then discussing with your clients use of the exercise for between-session practice. Form 9.6 has been modified to explore evidence for and against beliefs about the cause or origin of voices as well as the pros and cons of beliefs about the cause of voices. In addition, the pie chart (form 9.7) can be used to collaboratively explore explanations for voices.

Some psychoeducation about the potential explanations for voice hearing can be provided gently. These potential explanations may include, for example, voices as misattributed self-talk, including intrusive cognitions or dysfunctional attempts at thought suppression; difficulties with source monitoring or being able to accurately identify where a noise is coming from; and the tendency of those with a diagnosis of schizophrenia to have cognitive biases, including propensities toward jumping to conclusions and an externalizing bias (Bentall, 2004; Beck et al., 2009). Tape recording of the voice and checking with trusted others regarding whether they have heard a voice are other ways of collecting data about voices. Of course, any of these explanations and techniques for exploring voices must be dealt with using the utmost respect for your clients' voice hearing experience and culture and must be addressed from a stance of what is helpful versus what is not.

Relationship with Voices

Your clients' relationship with their voices is an extremely important piece of the understanding and approach to working with the voices. The purpose of the voice (compensatory, company, interest, valued other) was discussed earlier and is important to explore with your clients in depth. More adaptive ways of getting your clients' needs met should be explored and developed. Exploration of the adaptiveness of your clients' relationship with their voices is critical to address submissiveness and clients' past and typical response to command voices (see Byrne, Birchwood, Trower, & Meaden [2006], a case study book that includes a focus on a social rank theory understanding of voices). Critically, as emphasized in CFT, a focus on your clients shifting their relationship with their voices to one of compassion serves to deactivate the threat emotional system—CFT approaches to voices are key here. Of note, your clients' relationship with their voices is dynamic and should be explored throughout the therapy process to clarify and work with any changes as well as to enhance your clients' sense of power and control related to voices, including the ability to not act on command voices.

Culture

It is essential to address the cultural and spiritual contexts of the voices. You should enhance your understanding of your clients' culture, religion, and spirituality and how these may impact your clients' voice hearing experience and beliefs about voices. Inclusion of cultural, religious, and/or spiritual leaders or members can help to clarify whether the voice experience and related beliefs are consistent with the culture or religion. For example, a client who was hearing voices denigrating God was under the belief that she needed to engage in rituals of "forgiveness" for six to eight hours per day to demonstrate her devotion to God. When the client's priest was consulted (with the client's consent), it became clear that the client's actions were not consistent with her religion. By including her priest in the discussion of her voices and her responses to them, the client was able to spend less time engaging in her rituals and more time involved in her religious community. Given that it can be extremely difficult to work directly with distressing voices of a religious or spiritual nature or connection, it is possible to address them through the core beliefs (such as badness or worth) that may fuel them.

Core Belief or Schema Change

Therapeutic work with voices (and delusions) is intrinsically intertwined with the understanding of, and work with, core beliefs. Exploration of beliefs about denigrating voices, skill development, goal-directed activity, and almost all of the strategies discussed relate to, and are part of, the work on core beliefs. The experiential role play exercises with your clients (see the "Role Play and Exposure" section later in this chapter) can be very powerful in core belief change, as can the use of strategies such as writing an empowering letter to the voice. Chapter 4 highlights core beliefs and psychosis in the conceptualization and treatment planning process.

Command Voices

Therapeutic work with command hallucinations is critical, given the link with your clients' core beliefs, level of distress, and safety issues for them and others. Much of the work around command voices is focused on the relationship between your clients and the voices and in particular around the perceived power differential. Multiple cognitive behavioral strategies can be implemented, as described in previous sections). Behavioral experiments that challenge the power of the voice and the validity of the voice's threats are extremely helpful. Of note, you should be on the lookout for any appeasement behaviors that may get in the way of this work on the perceived power differential. For example, clients may do a behavioral experiment and, while not following through on what the voice says, may "appease" the voice by doing something else, such as hurting themselves in a lesser way by scraping rather than cutting their skin.

Coping Strategies Versus Unhelpful Behaviors

An often neglected area in therapeutic work with voices is the exploration of clients' existing coping strategies or ways of dealing with voices. Careful exploration of coping strategies reinforces a strengths-based and empowering approach to your clients and provides essential information. It is important to check out not only what strategies are used but when and for what reasons. (See Voice Diary, form 9.1; see also Coping Strategies for Voices, form 9.8, which is discussed below.) If clients use a strategy to avoid voices, they may actually increase anxiety and fear around the voice and not have the opportunity to develop coping strategies to deal with the voice—the result being that the strategy comes to serve an avoidance function. Safety behaviors can actually contribute to fear and disempowerment, and they can increase the experience of voices, again serving an avoidance function. Use of appeasement strategies (for example, putting a knife to the wrist but not cutting) can maintain or increase your clients' belief about the power of voices. An extensive list of coping strategies for voices is presented in form 9.8. Examples of some coping strategies listed include taping the voice or using coping cards, a voice buddy, ear phones, subvocalization, and so on. Consistent with the discussion above, it is important to distinguish coping versus avoidance in the use of these strategies so that they may be used by your clients in an adaptive and empowering manner. Earlier in this chapter the Voice Diary (form 9.1) was used as a log to assess and monitor voices; this form is useful to continue the exploration of voices and the adaptiveness of coping strategies.

Behavioral Experiments

As with delusions, the use of behavioral experiments (see form 9.9) can be very powerful in reducing fear and believability of voices. Before engaging in a behavioral experiment, it is critical to explore with your clients what it would mean if the experiment turned out one way versus the other. For example, the result could be explained away by clients saying things such as "You set it up" or "That wouldn't happen in real life." Behavioral experiments that can be very powerful are taping the voice or asking if others can hear the voice.

Role Play and Exposure

Role play using Socratic dialogue has multiple goals and benefits. Through role play, your clients can experientially establish a different, healthier relationship with their voices that cause distress. In addition, your clients can gain greater distance and objectivity in relation to their voices, and engage in a form of exposure that can increase self-efficacy and diminish fear and avoidance around voices. Role plays and two-chair work enhance emotion within session and enable your clients to develop their ability to cope with the emotions experienced as a result of the voices. These experiential exercises are also helpful in developing more self-compassion and shifting negative core beliefs.

Exposure (also called focusing) can be used with voices in a way similar to its use for anxiety and feared objects or situations. Role plays are used, as in other exposure approaches, in a graded manner to increase self-efficacy. In doing role plays with voices, your clients first role-play the least distressing or least threatening role. In example 1 below, you will demonstrate for your clients, responding constructively to their voice. In examples 2, 3, and 4, your clients will be given the experience, in session, of responding to the voice. Finally, as "homework" (example 5), your clients will respond to voices outside the session.

Example 1. You will role-play your clients, responding to their voice, and your clients role-play their voice. (You will demonstrate how to do this to your clients.)

Example 2. You role-play your clients' voice. Your clients role-play responding to the voice, but they do so as someone they care about or admire would. This more graded approach enables your clients to practice Socratic questioning and responding to the voice, but in a less personal and threatening way.

Example 3. Your client role-plays responding to the voice in session while you role-play being the voice.

Example 4. This is a modification of the above role play: an experiential two-chair method with voices (Greenberg, Greenley, McKee, Brown, & Griffin-Francell, 1993; Chadwick, 2006), as described below:

One chair is designated as the "voice chair," the other "voice response chair." Your clients alternate between role-playing the voice in the voice chair and responding to the voice from the voice response chair. Facilitate this process and then summarize the discussion from the chair exercise. You and your clients then explore together the experience, meaning, and implications of the chair method in understanding and having a more empowering response to the voice's derogatory content. Of course, the ultimate goal is to gradually start to shift your clients' negative core beliefs or schemas about themselves.

Example 5. As "homework," your clients dialogue with the voices outside the session in a private, safe place. To enhance a sense of mastery, it is essential that you and your clients have discussed the homework and the approach to the homework thoroughly. Clearly delineate in session (in writing) the best situations in which to do the exposure work, and problem-solve any challenges that might occur.

Of note, the distress level of the content of the voices is approached in a hierarchical manner in each of the progressive role plays above. Prior to initiating the role plays, you and your clients collaboratively develop the hierarchy based on the distress a client reports experiencing in response to his or her voices.

In addition to the graded exposure approach to voices above, it is possible to take a graded approach to exposure to situations associated with the voices. You and your clients complete the Voice Avoidance Hierarchy (form 9.10) together. Your client then works toward increasing distress exposure, thereby enhancing self-efficacy with voices and reducing avoidance and isolation.

Metacognitive Approaches

Metacognitive approaches have previously been discussed in the therapeutic work with distressing thoughts or delusions (see chapter 8). The same principles and approaches apply with voices. Your clients gain experience in thinking about their thinking, beliefs, or voices, to gain perspective and to notice any patterns, so that they can then try to act in a more workable or "adaptive" manner. The use of the form Pros and Cons of Time Focused on Voices (9.11) to check out the advantages and disadvantages of the time focused on voices rather than goal-directed activity can be very useful. Throughout the therapeutic work on voices, we emphasize an orientation toward acceptance of the potential of continuing to hear some voices over the "unworkable" struggle to permanently silence voices that often consumes so much time and energy.

Coping Cards

Coping cards can be a very effective tool to help clients deal with distressing voices. The coping card is completed collaboratively by you and your clients in session. Your clients generate "reasonable" thoughts or beliefs about their voices and/or ways of coping with the voices and record these on an index card, which then becomes a "coping card." It is critical that your clients record these thoughts, beliefs, and coping strategies in their own words on the coping card, as this enhances the validity of the statements. Your clients carry the coping card with them at all times and refer to it when they experience distressing voices. This strategy is like a form of cued self-coaching; it can help improve your clients' insight when they are distressed. The coping card can also be used as a way for clients to work on enhancing self-esteem and shifting core beliefs; they can generate and record personal qualities and accomplishments on the card. Despite the simplicity of this approach, the use of coping cards can be invaluable for many clients. Depending on your clients' preferences, you or your clients can write one or multiple coping statements on each card. Below are some examples of the types of statements that can be used on coping cards:

- My voice is just a voice. What it says is not based on facts.

- I am a good person. I don't deserve to be treated unkindly by my voices.

- My voice is just my own critical self-talk.

- My voice is not a threat to me. I do not need to act on my voice.

Voice Time

Just as allocating worry time each day can be an effective tool for dealing with anxiety, many clients find that designating a set amount of time to spend with their voices can reduce the intrusiveness, frequency, and duration of voices. Designated voice time can also enhance your clients' sense of their ability to impact voice hearing and be in the "driver's seat." Clients use various strategies to respond to their voices when they are present at times other than the time allocated for voices ("voice time"). While gentle redirection can be effective, many clients report that simply telling their voices that they will talk to them later works!

Attention Training

Due to a difficulty with source monitoring often found in those with psychosis who hear voices, attention training has been used to enhance source-monitoring skills related to voices. Those who hear voices are often found to have deficits in discriminating where stimuli originate as well as in screening out irrelevant stimuli. Therefore, subvocal self-talk, for example, can be misattributed to an external voice. To address this difficulty, the metacognitive therapy approach of attention training described by Wells (2000) involves a focus on five neutral auditory stimuli or noises in the room (for example, the hums of a refrigerator or heater, or a dripping tap), switching attention between different pairs of noises, and practicing the deployment of attention by listening to all the sounds at the same time. After some weeks of attentional practice and skill consolidation, the voice is introduced as "just" another sound. Your clients learn to switch their attention between the neutral sounds and their voice, then back and forth between the voice and other sounds, and then between the sounds and the voice. The recommended practice is for five to ten minutes twice daily, but this strategy should be tried out repeatedly in session before ongoing practice at home is attempted. Mindfulness exercises can also be used to enhance skills in noticing internal and external stimuli and taking a more distanced or metacognitive stance with thoughts, voices, and emotions.

Positive Memory Training

Van der Gaag, Nieman, & Van den Berg (2013) have developed an empirically supported approach to positive memory training for those who hear voices. To use this approach, collaboratively develop a positive memory image using all senses. Practice using this positive memory first in session and then as practice between sessions at least five times per day. Also develop a voice come-back or response that is practiced in session and out. Then pair the positive memory and voice come-back with the experience of voices.

More on Acceptance, Mindfulness, and Compassion-Focused Therapeutic Approaches

As previously discussed, acceptance, mindfulness, and compassion-focused approaches can be very enriching. In particular, an emphasis on acceptance that voices may continue and then focusing on helpful ways to cope with voices rather than "doing battle" with them can free up time and energy for meaningful pursuits. We have found that a focus on a shift in the relationship that our clients have with their voices can be very powerful. Making statements such as "Hello, voices" or "Thanks, voices" and then returning to goal-directed activity can—along with other strategies, and over time—develop a qualitatively different way of responding to and interacting with voices. The analogy of quicksand for the "struggle with voices" can help provide an image of how struggling can take us deeper and be counterproductive or even harmful to the pursuit of life goals and meaning.

Mindfulness can be used as a way of bringing our clients into contact with thoughts, physical sensations, emotions, and voices—and without judgment, as much as possible! By noticing voices through mindfulness approaches, experiential avoidance of voices is countered but in a safer, shorter (a few minutes), and supported context. Again, mindfulness shifts the relationship or approach to voices and provides distance or opportunity for defusion from the voices. Mindfulness is in and of itself an exposure exercise!

Compassion-focused exercises can focus on compassion for self and eventually compassion for the voices. By shifting the relationship with the voices, the power differential is implicitly addressed. Here are some examples of acceptance, mindfulness, and compassion-focused strategies for voices:

- Write a compassionate letter to self.

- Write a compassionate letter to voices (to shift the relationship with the voice).

- Do mindfulness of voices exercise.

- Create compassionate coping cards: a thought is just a thought; a voice is just a voice; compassionate responses to voices; compassionate responses to self when experiencing voices.

- Use a tug-of-war metaphor to highlight that struggling with voices can be exhausting and increase distress, whereas a more normalizing and accepting stance can be helpful in diminishing the distress associated with hearing voices.

- Utilize imagery such as leaves on a stream (putting the voices on leaves on a stream, and watching them drift away) to highlight the transitory nature of voices.

- Use the image of a volume knob to decrease voices or shut them off. The knob image can be helpful as can the ACT metaphor or idea of turning off the "struggle switch" in one's relationship with one's voices.

For more examples of acceptance, mindfulness, and compassion-focused strategies for voices, see the list in Coping Strategies for Voices (form 9.8).

Action Plan

As previously indicated, the goal in working therapeutically with voices is a reduction in distress, enhanced functioning, meaningful value-directed activity, and committed action. All of the above shifts can lead to a fuller and more meaningful life. For example, voices may not change in frequency and loudness, but if the conviction in the content of distressing voices shifts, your clients' experience of voices shifts in a life- and self-affirming manner.

Due to the episodic, often recurring nature of some psychotic symptoms, it is essential to work on developing a wellness or action plan for voices that proactively identifies stressors, triggers, and coping strategies, thereby reducing the likelihood of relapse and demoralization. A caution here: Clients may become hypervigilant to warning signs and triggers due to fears about "relapse" or a recurrence of voices. A heightened vigilance and selective attention to certain physical experiences and perceived threats may increase stress and generate "false positives." Acceptance- and mindfulness-based understandings and approaches can be helpful in these cases. For an example of a wellness action plan for voices, see form 9.12. An activity schedule and work toward increased goal-directed activity can be very helpful for addressing negative symptoms and committed action.

Between-Session Practice

Collaboratively decide on the between-session practice, clarify understanding, and problem-solve any potential barriers to practice. Give example handouts or worksheets to your client as well as corresponding blank handouts or worksheets to fill out.

Feedback from Client on the Session

Solicit feedback from your client during and at the end of each session. Feedback is particularly important with work with voices as clients have often been discounted or not felt safe or comfortable enough to be able to discuss their voice hearing experiences.

Summary of Session

Collaboratively fill in the Session Summary (form 5.1) with your clients. Ask your clients to read the psychoeducation handouts and share this information with their family, friends, and caregivers. Continue to model a focus on strengths, qualities, and/or accomplishments by generating examples from the session.

Coping Exercise (Optional)

See forms 4.2 and 9.8 in the appendix for a selection of coping exercises.

Additional Resources

For more information, please see the Resources section of this book. You will find many of the forms in the appendix; they are also available for download at http://www.newharbinger.com/24076. (See the back of this book for instructions on how to access them.) Additional materials not available in this book can be found on our website at http://www.treatingpsychosis.com.

CHAPTER 10

Module 7: Accomplishments and Staying Well Plan— Ongoing Recovery, Valued Life Goals, and Staying Well

This module on accomplishments, progress, and staying well can be broken down into therapy sessions based on client needs. A written staying well plan that highlights achievements, strengths, and coping strategies as well as warning signs, triggers, and a step-by-step action plan focused on emotion regulation within the context of a strengths-focused approach is essential to maintaining ongoing well-being and living a full and meaningful life.

Materials

See appendix for forms. They are also available for download at http://www.newharbinger.com/24076. (See the back of this book for instructions on how to access them.)

Form 10.1 Staying Well Plan

Modifications for Group Implementation

Although coping skills, strengths, resources, and staying well are emphasized throughout the therapy group, the last few sessions focus on consolidation of gains made, future plans, and, in particular, the development of a personal written staying well plan. Your client's strengths, coping strategies, and resources list (form 4.3) should be revisited in group and shared with group members. The staying well module also gives group participants the opportunity to provide feedback to other group members of changes or progress they have noticed and things they have valued in having each person in the group. Group members will often want to keep in touch with one another. This can be done through booster sessions scheduled by the group leaders (perhaps monthly) or an open group that can be offered weekly or biweekly on an ongoing basis for anyone who participated in the group over the past number of years. If group members wish to share contact information, this is supported. However, some group members may not wish to remain in contact with other group members; therefore, an assumption should not be made regarding the sharing of contact information. Evaluation measures and feedback forms can be filled out in the last session prior to celebrating the completion of the group. (See our website http://www.treatingpsychosis.com for a list of relevant evaluation measures.) Blank envelopes for completed questionnaires should be given to clients to ensure confidentiality. Alternatively, group leaders can meet individually with each group member after completion of the group to reinforce gains, problem-solve any issues in the staying well plan, schedule follow-up meetings, receive feedback, and complete any postgroup measures.

Goals and Outline of Module (1 to 3 sessions)

Refer to the resources on the companion website (http://www.treatingpsychosis.com). Using form 4.3, a complete list of your clients' strengths, coping strategies, and resources should have been compiled on an ongoing basis by you and your clients. Bring the consolidated strengths list to the sessions on accomplishments and the staying well plan. Add to the strengths list as ideas come up. The strengths list is an integral part of the staying well plan. The focus in relapse prevention as emphasized throughout the integrated treatment is on ongoing use of coping skills, work toward valued goals, and targeting emotion dysregulation through enhancing emotion regulation and emotional resilience.

Agenda for the Session

Collaboratively decide with your clients what you would like to address in the staying well sessions. Start first with accomplishments and consolidation of progress made, including emotion regulation strategies developed and found to be helpful to cope with distressing emotions.

Check-In

Complete a check-in with your clients based on their functioning since the last session, including the day of the current session. The check-in can involve the following ratings:

Mood rating 0–10 (10 being the highest level of positive mood)

Anxiety rating 0–10 (10 being the highest level of anxiety)

Self-efficacy or accomplishment rating 0–10 (10 being the highest level of self-efficacy or accomplishment)

Psychosis rating 0–10 (10 constituting the highest level of distress associated with thoughts, delusions, and/or hallucinations, such as voices). A number of different ratings for voices can be used such as believability/conviction, control, power, frequency, and disruption of clients' work toward meaningful goals.

Summary and Link to Previous Sessions

Ask your clients what they recall from the last session. Reinforce what was recalled and/or normalize difficulties with remembering material from session to session. Summarize the material from the previous session and link it to the between-session practice and the session's topic. When discussing accomplishments and the staying well plan, a review of the material and skills covered over the course of the treatment should be conducted and cross-referenced with the strengths, coping strategies, and resources list (form 4.3).

Review and Problem-Solving of Between-Session Practice

Ask your clients about their experience with doing the between-session practice. Reinforce what was completed. Empathetically normalize any difficulties your clients had with the practice. Collaboratively problem-solve any of the barriers or difficulties raised. Remind your clients that after treatment is finished, it will be important for them to identify and problem-solve barriers to practice and staying well in their day-to-day life.

Coping Exercise

Give your clients a list with descriptions/instructions of all of the coping exercises (see form 4.2) that you have tried in the treatment sessions and at home. Discuss your clients' plans for ongoing incorporation of the coping strategies in their daily life. Proactively problem-solve any potential barriers or challenges to implementing coping strategies. Develop a plan for addressing difficulties with use of coping strategies after completion of therapy (booster follow-up sessions, support from caregivers/family, books or web-based instructions, and so on). It can be helpful for you and your clients to put coping skills on the Activity Form (form 7.2).

Overview of Session/Topic Area for Clients

Provide a brief overview of the importance of consolidating progress and accomplishments as well as developing and implementing a staying well plan. It is important to emphasize a focus on ongoing wellness without contributing to or creating a fear of relapse that could involve elevated vigilance for changes in physiological sensations, emotions, or experiences.

Clinician Stance

Your stance should be one of encouragement and reinforcement around progress made and plans for staying well. The feel of these sessions should be one of celebration, pride, and recognizing accomplishments and movement toward meaningful goals and living a value-consistent life.

Module Therapeutic Strategies and Exercises

This module contains information and approaches for the staying well plan, as described below. (For more information and strategies for relapse prevention, see Copeland, 2010; Gumley & Schwannauer, 2006; and Gumley, Gillham, Taylor, & Schwannauer, 2013.) Consistent with the research literature (see Gumley et al., 2013), the focus for staying well and relapse prevention is continued implementation of coping strategies with a focus on the psychological processes and mechanisms associated with emotion regulation and resiliency. Given the (understandable) fear of relapse in psychosis, there can be catastrophic expectations and fears of setbacks or relapse and resulting hypervigilance and sensitivity. In addition, delays in seeking help can arise due to fears of relapse and avoidance of dealing with fears and threats of relapse.

Complete the staying well plan collaboratively with your clients. It will be important to be aware of the triggering of negative beliefs about relapse and about self, others, and the illness. When identifying early signs, a focus on shifting beliefs to a more internal locus of control by enhancing your clients' sense of self-efficacy and agency and discussing the ability to address factors under their control is beneficial. Focus on enhancing a sense of mastery and coping skills. Also, exploration of both the evidence for and against the likelihood of relapse and the more catastrophic beliefs regarding relapse is essential. Work on the identification of false alarms can reduce stress and can enhance targeting of efforts. Relapse prevention and staying well are ongoing parts of the engagement, assessment, and treatment process, rather that something that is addressed solely at the end of treatment. The next two sections can be used as guides for presenting a wellness plan to clients.

Client Information: Staying Well

It is important for all of us to do things on a daily basis to stay healthy and well. We will be discussing these staying well tools as well as early warning signs and triggers as part of developing a personal "staying well plan." The staying well plan is like a "plan of action," and it includes staying well tools and activities as well as the knowledge of signs that may indicate that we are not doing as well. Important things we can all do for ourselves include eating well; getting enough sleep; exercising; reducing caffeine; talking to friends, family, and health care providers to get support and help; taking prescribed medication regularly; reducing or stopping the use of alcohol and street drugs; reducing or quitting smoking; and adopting other healthy habits. We have discussed coping exercises such as relaxation, imagery, deep breathing, perspective taking, coping cards, and so on. To stay well, it is important to keep on using these coping exercises on a regular basis—every day! Just like when we are trying to get more healthy and lose weight, we can't just change what we do for one day but need to keep at it regularly. List strategies you can use as part of your staying well plan on form 10.1.

Client Information: Triggers and Early Warning Signs

Even if we do all we can to stay well, we can have stresses or setbacks sometimes. Stressors, or *triggers*, can be things like an illness, a change in school or work, an anniversary, and so on. And stressors may increase the likelihood of relapse. Knowing what your triggers are can be helpful to make sure to take extra care and get help, if needed. Helpful ways to deal with triggers can be to make an appointment with your doctor, talk to a friend, take a rest and relaxation day, or do other things that are good for you. Write your ways of coping with triggers in your staying well plan (form 10.1).

In addition to triggers, there can be *early warning signs*—signals that we may be starting to become unwell. With early warning signs, it's important (1) to know that setbacks may happen, (2) to notice your early warning signs, and (3) to have a plan to deal with those early warning signs. Here are some common early warning signs:

- poor sleep

- an increase in symptoms (for example, more voices, more paranoia, confused thinking, and so on)

- poor eating habits

- withdrawing from others

- feeling more anxious

- feeling more fearful

- feeling more down

- thinking and feeling like you can't cope

- feeling helpless

- feeling hopeless

- reduced concentration

- less interest in activities

- increased irritability

- experiences like being more sensitive or suspicious in social situations; hearing voices or more distressing voices; experiencing changes in thinking and changes in what you notice, such as what you see, hear, feel, smell, or taste.

Use form 10.1 to list your early warning signs to help you with your staying well plan. Remember to keep your strengths, coping strategies, and resources list (form 4.3) close at hand so you can remind yourself of your strengths, qualities, and accomplishments as well as of the coping strategies and resources that you have.

Feedback from Client on the Session

Solicit feedback from your clients during and at the end of the session as well as the treatment as a whole and the staying well plan. Ask your clients to complete a treatment satisfaction measure and outcome evaluation measures. (See http://www.treatingpsychosis.com for examples.)

Summary of Progress, Staying Well Plan, and Staying Well Tune-Up Sessions

Ask your clients to share the summary of accomplishments and strengths as well as the staying well plan with family, friends, or caregivers, if they want to. Make an appointment for a staying well tune-up session with your clients, or discuss follow-up and make an appointment with the follow-up service provider (including information about the treatment program, the staying well plan, and the list of the client's accomplishments and strengths). Highlight progress and indicate that the journey of life naturally involves some bumps along the way, but that your clients have tools to use to cope with the bumps and to continue to grow and create a meaningful life and future.

Celebration

Celebrate your clients, their progress, strengths, and qualities. Providing a certificate of achievement (for groups) or asking your clients how they would like to acknowledge and celebrate what they have achieved can be very powerful. Providing a verbal and written summary of progress, skills, and qualities can enhance internalization of a sense of achievement.

Additional Resources

For more information, please see the Resources section of this book. You will find many of the forms in the appendix; they are also available for download at http://www.newharbinger.com/24076. (See the back of this book for instructions on how to access them.) Additional materials not available in this book can be found on our website at http://www.treatingpsychosis.com.

PART 3

FURTHER
CONSIDERATIONS

CHAPTER 11

Special Considerations
and Comorbidity

It has not been possible to fully address particular clinical populations, situations, and issues that are important for consideration. Although most of the topics outlined below are addressed through our integrated trauma-informed approach to conceptualization, engagement, assessment, and treatment, we wish to highlight areas for special consideration and refer the reader to additional resources for further information. This list is by no means exhaustive. We have written additional papers on a number of these topics to provide more in-depth information regarding theory, research, assessment, and treatment. These papers are available on our website http://www.treatingpsychosis.com. Other resources are noted in the Resources section of this book.

Trauma and Post-Traumatic Stress Disorder

Given the extremely high level of trauma histories and experiences in those with lived experience of psychosis, we have written a paper on trauma and PTSD in psychosis that gives an overview of the research literature, treatment approaches, and resources. We emphasize that a trauma-informed approach is crucial from initial assessment through each stage of intervention, given the prevalence of trauma in the histories of individuals presenting with psychosis, the trauma that can be experienced related to the symptoms of psychosis, the trauma that can occur through coming into contact with the justice or health care system, and the trauma that can be experienced as a result of the risks associated with poverty and marginalization.

Comorbid Anxiety Problems/Disorders

Although the principles for treatment of psychosis and anxiety are the same, we also offer on our website a paper and additional resources on anxiety problems and disorders most commonly experienced in those with psychosis, including general anxiety or worry, social anxiety, obsessive-compulsive disorder or problems with obsessions and compulsion, and panic. Consideration of anxiety and comorbid anxious conditions is critical. We highlight the role of such areas as selective attention to threat, hypervigilance, overestimating the probability of risk, avoidance-oriented strategies such as worry and rumination (rather than active coping strategies), intrusions and their link with voices and fears around mind reading, compulsions associated with intrusive thoughts and misinterpretation, or catastrophic interpretations of physiological sensations. In addition, we discuss individual and group treatment for anxiety, including group-based treatment interventions that we have developed and implemented with those with psychosis for general anxiety disorder (GAD), social anxiety, OCD, and emotion regulation.

Substance Use

Substance use is a common problem occurring in people who experience psychosis for multiple reasons. The research literature supports an integrated treatment approach to working with psychosis and substance use in which the same team or clinicians address the issues around both. The theory, principles, and treatment strategies we have included in this guide address both psychosis and substance use by focusing on values and goals as well as employing adaptive strategies to address the function or purpose that substances play in the individual's life. See the Resources section and our website, http://www.treatingpsychosis.com for more information.

Early Psychosis/First Episode

At the time of the first episode, it is crucial to have CBT delivered as early as possible, ideally at the prodrome stage. Morrison et al. (2012) have shown that delivering CBT to people with prodromes results in reduced severity of symptoms at the time of onset of the first episode. Research has been conducted on those at high risk for psychosis that speaks to the importance of early recognition, support, and resources during schooling and in primary care. The integrated treatment model and approaches presented in this guide have been designed to be suitable for first episode psychosis. However, further emphasis on peers, families, developmental issues, and the role of substance use is important. Please refer to French and

Morrison (2004) for a treatment guide as well as our Resources section for further information on special considerations and modifications in those with early psychosis.

Considerations for Forensics and Corrections Settings

Unfortunately, some clients with psychosis may come into contact with the law and be served within a forensic (mental health) or corrections setting. As levels of trauma within the forensic and corrections populations are extremely high, a trauma-informed approach is essential. As in other settings, a caring and compassionate, destigmatizing approach that is strengths- and empowerment-oriented is key. Therapy can be somewhat more difficult for these clients due to their fears of disclosing information to clinicians and the implications this may have for them. Risk, as with others with psychosis, should be targeted. Again, working with clients on the omnipotence and omniscience of the voice using an approach based in social rank theory is advisable (see Byrne et al., 2007; Tarrier et al., 2013). Clients may be dealing with feelings of guilt or remorse over the "offense," which can feed into negative symptoms and internalized stigma. Often clients have not had the opportunity to review all the evidence surrounding the case. If given a chance to do this (for example, in a courtroom role play), they might develop greater understanding of why they acted in the way they did, thereby facilitating a greater sense of self-forgiveness. Stigma (and self-stigma) are critical pieces to address with all individuals with psychosis, but may be even more of an issue within forensic and correctional settings. Consistent with our integrated model and approach, a nonjudgmental, compassionate, and empowering approach can enhance quality of life and recovery.

Community-Based Treatment

Treatment is often most effective when practiced within clients' own homes or communities, where they will usually feel safer and more comfortable. This also gives the opportunity to do reality testing experiments and to practice coping strategies more easily. Assertive community treatment teams can implement and reinforce many of the approaches in our treatment. We have provided approaches both in this guide and on our website that can be implemented more easily when time constraints are an issue—ten-minute approaches, for example. See the resources section of http://www.treatingpsychosis. com for a list of books that offer brief approaches for CBT, mindfulness, and stress.

Family and Caregivers

Family, friends, and caregivers are in an excellent position to support clients and the therapy work of their clinicians. Ideally, family should be involved as much as possible to support those with psychosis and their progress. Psychoeducation is a critical piece of work with families. In particular, an understanding, nonjudgmental environment and approach that focuses on strengths is important for supporting clients to work toward valued goals and staying well. The family and/or caregivers should have an understanding of the factors that trigger, perpetuate, maintain, and protect against distressing psychosis. In addition, depending on the wishes of the client, family members can reinforce and assist clients with practice and homework. Family and caregiver involvement in relapse prevention or staying well is crucial. This includes, as much as possible, being involved in developing and supporting the client's staying well plan. Care for the caregiver is essential. See the Resources section for information and support for families—for example, the National Alliance on Mental Illness (NAMI), the local Schizophrenia Society, *The Complete Family Guide to Schizophrenia* by Mueser and Gingerich (2006), and so on. Family psychoeducation and support, and therapy done on an individual or multifamily group basis, can be an important adjunct to treatment for clients. Research on family groups for psychosis notes the benefits of multifamily group interventions as a complement to treatment for clients with psychosis (see McFarlane, 2002).

Stigma

Those with lived experience of psychosis indicate that they struggle not only with psychotic symptoms but also with the label of schizophrenia. Clients often struggle with both the stigma and perceived stigma associated with a diagnosis of schizophrenia. They also struggle with self-stigma, which involves internalizing perceived stigma or negative stereotyping and prejudice associated with having a mental illness. Self-stigma and the accuracy of thoughts and beliefs around societal stigma are explored throughout the treatment. Clients can often detect distressing thoughts relating to self-worth, "brain damage," being labeled "crazy," and fears around potential hospitalization. In addition, given the media coverage around risk and psychosis, stigma around others' perceptions of the risk of violence can be an issue. Therapeutic work with shame-based, denigrating, and self-critical thoughts is implicitly and explictly addressed in our strengths-focused, positive psychology–infused treatment approach. Therapeutic work around self-identity and self-valuing is an integral part of the work around distressing thoughts and voices as well as actual and perceived stigma and judgment by others. Often these stigma-flavored thoughts are represented by an image. Such mental imagery can be laden with affect. Clinicians can work with clients' thoughts and images to minimize self-stigma and enhance more whole, humanistic, and empowered beliefs about self. Unfortunately, because clients can be the subject of stigma in everyday life and in the sensationalist media, psychoeducation of clients, families, caregivers, health professionals, and the public is crucial.

CBT for Clients with Thought Disorders or Severe Cognitive Deficits

Clients who experience a milder degree of disorganization of thought can engage in therapeutic work by adding the techniques of thought linkage, thematic analysis, and a focus on the theme driving the thought disorder (for example, hurt, anxiety, or anger). If acceptable, sessions can be videotaped, as review can reveal important triggers for affective change and change in body posture. Sessions need to be brief and tend to be more tiring than normal sessions. Treatment should be tailored for level of cognitive function. Suggestions for treatment individualization are addressed throughout this guide. In addition, we have included simplified versions of forms on the New Harbinger website (http://www .newharbinger.com/24076). For more information on this area and for examples of cognitive remediation programs, see Wykes & Reeder (2005) and Wykes et al. (2012).

Risk

The importance of assessing and addressing risk in those who experience psychosis cannot be overemphasized. Throughout our treatment guide, we have emphasized the importance of addressing risk, including thoughts of harm to self and others, as a primary focus for assessment and intervention. The assessment form (4.1) addresses risk, and chapter 9 addresses the potential risk associated with command hallucinations and strategies for reducing compliance with command hallucinations. See Tarrier and colleagues (2013) for their treatment manual on CBT prevention of suicide in psychosis, and Meaden, Keen, Aston, Barton, and Bucci (2013) for their advanced practical companion on cognitive therapy for command hallucinations. Given the distressing nature of psychosis, thoughts of harm to self can arise with many clients. An openness on the part of the clinician to discussing clients' thoughts of harm to self, due to feeling overwhelmed and hopeless, should be acknowledged and explored. This should be done with an extremely caring (and comprehensive) approach to risk assessment, development of an associated safety plan, as well as enhancement of clients' sense of meaning, power, control, and self.

CBT and Adherence

Adherence with antipsychotic medication regimes has been an area of interest. Antipsychotics remain the mainstay of treatment for most clients experiencing distressing thoughts, delusions, voices, and negative symptoms. However, adherence is often very poor, and partial adherence is the rule rather than the exception. There is one "delusion" that we know to be true: we as health care professionals and psychiatrists can mistakenly believe that our clients adhere well to prescribed medicines. The issue of partial adherence is extremely problematic as it leads to intermittent receptor blockade, which can set a client up for relapse via the mechanism of episodic receptor hypersensitivity to stress or hallucinogens.

Why do clients not adhere? The answer is simple: adherence is difficult under the best circumstances. Early on, clients need very clear information about what the medicine does and how long they will be required to take it. The National Institute for Health and Care Excellence (2009) states that once in a state of recovery, a client could begin a supervised gradual reduction of antipsychotic medications after two years. That supervision would ideally be done by a psychiatrist and a CBT therapist who could help the client with the anxiety symptoms, distressing thoughts, and intrusions that can appear as medication is reduced. Cultural aspects are also important, with many cultures not endorsing biological models of psychosis and therefore opting for traditional faith-related remedies. Try traditional approaches first, if it is safe to do so, in the hope of scientific evaluation of any benefits or problems.

Lack of insight is another major factor. Indeed, Rathod, Kingdon, Smith, and Turkington (2005) have argued that CBT mostly works via the vehicle of improved insight into the benefits of medication and via reality testing of psychotic experiences. Automatic thoughts can interfere with adherence and can be linked to underlying personal or family rules about medication. These can be detected and worked with. Values and valued goals, as identified and worked with in our integrated model, can be linked to medication adherence. Partnership prescribing allows the client to choose the side effect profile that would be least troublesome and can enhance adherence reporting.

Many clients refuse medication, whether for reasons of side effects (including weight gain), stigma, lack of insight, or personal preference. There is some early evidence that clients who refuse medication will engage in the offer of a "talking treatment." When CBT has been offered to those who refuse medication, it has been shown to be safe and acceptable and to deliver symptomatic benefit (Morrison et al., 2012). A small percentage of these clients opted to eventually begin antipsychotic medication after the CBT had finished. Further information on CBT for adherence to antipsychotics can be found in Weiden and Turkington (2012).

*

We hope you've found the approaches, issues, and possibilities addressed in this guide and in this special considerations section helpful. We also hope this guide will spur your interest in seeking more information in order to enrich your understanding and work with those who experience psychosis.

CHAPTER 12

Some Final Thoughts

The treatment plan we've presented in this book can help individuals affected by psychosis to live more goal-directed and fulfilling lives. Our approach relies on a deep and sincere compassion for clients and their experiences. We believe in establishing a warm, collaborative, and empowering therapeutic relationship with clients. Since psychotic symptoms exist along a continuum, we believe that symptoms need be addressed only to the extent that they cause distress to the client and interfere with life goals such as fulfilling relationships; satisfying educational, vocational, recreational, and employment activities; and engaging meaningfully with the community. We find that this compassionate, value-driven stance reduces stigma and helps clients feel safer in therapy, which in turn can allow for greater progress in treatment. We encourage you to try this approach, even if it seems unfamiliar at first, and see if the same is true for you and your clients.

Once you and your clients have worked together to clarify the clients' values and goals, you have a solid, shared foundation for exploring ways to regulate emotions; build resilience; cope with symptoms, including distressing thoughts, delusions, and voices; and handle challenges such as trauma, anxiety, and dissociation. By continually returning to your clients' values, you communicate your fundamental respect for your clients, and repeatedly underscore the reasons to work toward a better life, even when it is challenging to do so.

Our deepest wish is to improve the lives of those who experience psychosis and allow them to reach their full potential. We sincerely hope this book helps you as you work with your clients to reduce their suffering and help them live fuller and more meaningful lives.

Appendix: Forms

FORM 4.1:   Areas to Cover in Assessment

(Modified with permission from Beck et al., 2009)

A positive CBT therapy approach entails strengths-based meaning making. The approach involves an assessment of positive functioning. It is competency oriented and solution focused, and emphasizes current coping and skills as well as skill development. This approach is implicitly encouraging and reinforcing, and it involves constructive reframing and the instillation of hope as well as the pursuit of meaning and purpose.

A way of modeling and encouraging this positive orientation is to ask your clients to give a positive introduction of themselves or write out a strengths-based life history.

The VIA strengths questionnaire is an excellent clinical tool (see http://www.viacharacter.org). This inventory of character strengths and values in action can be a useful tool (see Peterson & Seligman, 2004).

Interview Data

Date(s) of interview

Name of interviewer

Site of interview

Source of referral

Reason for referral

Current General Client Information

Name

Date of birth/age

Gender

Marital/relationship status; duration of current status

Sexual orientation

Race

Ethnicity

Indigenous heritage

Native origin

Socioeconomic status/financial support

Occupation/vocation

Grade in school (if student)

Telephone numbers; degree of confidentiality available for messages at each number

Home address

Work address/information

Housing situation (e.g., house, apartment, rooming house, parents' house, shelter, no fixed address)

Occupants of dwelling, safety/health issues re housing, stability of housing

Social contacts: frequency, duration, quality, closeness

Current Personal Data

Interests

Religion

Needs/wishes

Current valued life goals

Values: examples of values include:

- Creativity, curiosity, judgment, openness, love of learning, wisdom
- Bravery, perseverance, honesty, zest
- Capacity to love and be loved, kindness, social involvement
- Teamwork, fairness, leadership
- Forgiveness, modesty, humility, carefulness, self-control
- Appreciation, gratitude
- Hope, optimism
- Humor and playfulness

Personal qualities (e.g., resilience, determination, courage)

Accomplishments (e.g., education, volunteer work, hero in dealing with health issues, inspiration in coping with difficulties)

Accomplishment memories

Best/positive memories

Supports

Resources

Weaknesses/vulnerabilities

Social interaction style

Stressors

General activity schedule (typical day in week)

Contentment/quality of life: examples of quality of life areas to cover include the following (see Snyder & Lopez, 2002):

- Sense of self, core belief regarding self
- Goals
- Values
- Health
- Financial
- Volunteer work
- Recreational—sports, hobbies, leisure, learning, creativity, helping, spiritual, religious, love, friends, family, children, home, neighborhood, community
- Resources
- Attachment, love, nurturance, primary support group, connectedness, empathic relationships, education opportunities and support, meaningful work, volunteering, self-efficacy, safe housing, sufficient income
- Access to quality health services and reliable health care

Contribution to society and the psychosocial environment

Main Concerns

History of main concerns

Symptoms/distressing experiences: type, frequency, duration, severity, distress, consequences, beliefs

Content/meaning of symptoms/experiences

Interaction/co-occurrence of symptoms/experiences

Eliciting situations/triggers/mediators

Reaction/coping strategies

Current other stressors/events of prior week

Onset of first occurrence: time, events, initial reaction, meaning/understanding

Beliefs formed in first episode and development/reinforcement

Premorbid beliefs

Stressors/trauma associated with first experience

Review of symptoms (current and past): hallucinations (all modalities); delusions (all classes); depressive episodes; manic episodes; panic attacks; phobias; obsessions; compulsions; intrusions/avoidance of traumatic memories; eating problems; sexual concerns; thoughts, plans, and attempts of harm to self, including suicidal thoughts (collaboratively explore reasons to live and develop safety plan); thoughts of harm to others, plans, attempts or acts of harm to others (collaboratively develop safety plan); command hallucinations re harm to self or others (ability to refuse commands, appeasement behaviors re commands); attentional problems; other emotional concerns.

- Appropriateness for therapy, including potential benefits and barriers
- How psychoses initially developed, including psychological vulnerability, interpersonal themes, and proximal events
- Predelusional belief system (e.g., religion, sexuality)
- Complexity of distressing delusions/voices (e.g., content, dimensions, conviction, frequency, loudness, pervasiveness)
- Meaning made of psychoses/experiences; attitudes toward distressing delusions/voices; self-concept regarding psychoses
- Situations where distressing delusions/voices increase/decrease, including antecedents/triggers (Using this information your clients can gain a greater sense of agency or control in relation to their experiences.)
- Consequences of psychoses, including potential costs and maintaining factors (e.g., distressing thoughts or delusions related to the CIA can make a person feel important; voices may serve as company for those who are isolated; "grandiose" thoughts, beliefs, or delusions can serve a compensatory function such as enhancing self-esteem, their reduction can leave a sense of loss or impact on sense of self-worth if other aspects of the self are not developed prior to or during work with these beliefs)

An exploration of the 4 Ps is important:

1. Predisposing factors (genetics, trauma)
2. Precipitating factors (e.g., stressor such as sexual abuse and stressors, reminders)
3. Perpetuating factors (e.g., smoking weed)
4. Protective factors (e.g., supportive family and caregivers)

Health Habits

Illicit substance use (current and past): Type, onset, last use, frequency/amount (current and at time of maximum use), reasons for use, effects (including effects on symptoms), need for higher doses, withdrawal effects, attempts to discontinue, legal and social effects (including parental and other relationships)

Nicotine use: amount

Caffeine use: amount, latest use in a typical day

Diet (e.g., healthy, diabetic, vegan/vegetarian, weight reduction, motivators and barriers such as financial; assess knowledge and resources regarding healthy weight)

Exercise: type, frequency, barriers/motivators

Sleep: total hours, pattern, difficulties (apnea, trauma history, insomnia—current interventions regarding the same)

Safety: housing, street involvement, marginalization, gang involvement, related to drug use

Physical Health

Height/weight

Allergies to medications

Illnesses, injuries, surgeries, and limitations (present and past)

Physical review of systems (present and past): seizures; loss of consciousness; major head injury; hypertension; diabetes; stroke; hypercholesterolemia; cancer; HIV; history of chemical exposure; and neurological, cardiac, pulmonary, gastrointestinal, hepatic, renal, thyroid, or hormonal problems (emphasis on cardiovascular health and diabetes due to potential side effects of medications)

Current Treatment

Current medications: name, purpose, dose, frequency, duration (at current dose and total usage), side effects, effectiveness

Current therapy, programs, groups, self-help books, coping strategies—client's perception of benefits/drawbacks, response, and participation

Psychiatric/psychotherapeutic treatment history (emphasis on what was helpful and not helpful, experience of treatment, progress, and use of treatment strategies)

Date (onset, completion)

Circumstances at onset (including thoughts, emotions, behaviors, substance use)

Circumstances of obtaining treatment (e.g., voluntary, involuntary, coercion and/or distress associated with same)

Name of treatment personnel or institution (psychiatrist, psychologist, therapist/clinician, hospital, day program)

Diagnoses

Treatment type (e.g., individual or group psychotherapy, medications, ECT)

Effectiveness—client's perception; interviewer's perception

Benefits and drawbacks

Family Psychiatric History

Relation to client (including side of family)

Condition (diagnosis; if unavailable, symptoms)

Basis for diagnosis (e.g., professional, suspected by client)

Treatments (psychotherapy, hospitalizations, medications)

Personal/Social History

Parents: age, ethnic background, health; if deceased—age, year, and cause of death

Siblings: age, gender, health; if deceased—age, year, and cause of death

Pregnancy/birth complications

Early development (any knowledge of delayed walking/talking)

Childhood (in general): quality of family relationships; religious upbringing; values or rituals

Residences

School: performance, strengths and difficulties, motivation, final education level

Friends (e.g., none, a few, many, a group, quality of friendships)

Intimate relationships (including engagements/marriages/divorces)

Children: gender, age, quality of relationships, frequency of contact

Occupations: type, maximum duration, most recent, reasons for termination

Military service: branch, years, combat exposure, type of discharge

Forensic contacts (e.g., arrests, convictions, incarcerations, parole, probation)

Major events/traumas (e.g., assault; bullying; abuse—sexual, physical, psychological/emotional; neglect; forced treatment; best/worst memories; influences); coping strategies for trauma

Current and past life goals

Attitude Toward Treatment

Goals for treatment

Problem list

Motivation for change; motivational enhancers

Expectations regarding therapy

Views/beliefs about medication

Beliefs about treatment and mental health problems/issues

Supports and barriers to treatment

Current Coping Strategies

Family, access, personal strengths and qualities, resources, literacy

Suitability for treatment:

Interest; motivation; optimism regarding therapy

Personal responsibility for change

Client goals

Alliance potential

Awareness, accessibility, and differentiation of thoughts and emotions (emotion granulation)

Observations

Appearance

Alertness

Psychomotor activity

Affect

Attention/interactiveness/eye contact

Speech

Thought processes

Orientation

General cognition/intelligence

Insight

Judgment

Risk

It is absolutely critical to address risk in the first session and subsequent sessions and to explore content, beliefs, and responses to command hallucinations (see Tarrier et al., 2013). In addition, it is essential to collaboratively develop a safety plan and share this with family, friends, treatment team, and appropriate others.

Suicidal ideation: thoughts, plan, means, previous attempts, family/other history of suicide attempts, reasons to live/hope, function of suicidal ideation, alternatives strategies to cope

Self-harm: cutting, appeasement behaviors, safety behaviors

Harm to others: explore command hallucinations, delusional beliefs

Safety: housing safety, substance use

Safety plan: for self and others

FORM 4.2: Coping Exercises

Here are some coping exercises that you can use throughout the day. More coping exercises and longer, guided versions of the coping exercises below can be found on our website at http://www.treating psychosis.com.

A Thought Is Just a Thought

- Think of thoughts as guesses or just words, not facts. Thoughts can be noticed (catch it) and let pass without judgment. Images, such as thoughts coming and going like gentle waves on the ocean, can be helpful.

Awareness Exercise for Distressing Thoughts or Voices

- Notice or "catch" thoughts, emotions, voices, or bodily sensations. Now label the thought, emotion, or experience. For example, *I just had a sad thought. I just had an angry thought about the voices.* Just notice the thought or sensation and gently let it go. Notice that thoughts, experiences, or sensations don't last—they come and go.

Belly Breathing

- "Belly" breathing—also known as diaphragmatic or "deep" breathing—is a helpful strategy you can use throughout the day. Take a deep belly breath. Inhale to the count of four, and then exhale for a longer time than your inhale—perhaps to the count of five. Pause after your exhale and then repeat. If this is stressful at first, focus on your slowed breathing, doing a longer exhale than inhale. A calming image or word such as "peace" or "relax" can be helpful to use.

Body Scan

- Notice your body from feet to head. Notice any areas of tension or discomfort. Let go of any tension. The body scan can be used for a few moments or minutes multiple times each day to catch and let go of tension you carry in your body. (For a longer, guided body scan, go to http://www.treatingpsychosis.com.)

Coping Affirmations

- Think of healthy and helpful statements about yourself, your accomplishments, your strengths, and your qualities. Write the coping statements or affirmations on a coping card that you can look at whenever you want. (You can put the coping card in your wallet or purse or on a wall.) Practice saying the affirmations. You can make it like a new habit over time. These statements can shift unhealthy or unhelpful beliefs. (You can also use coping strategies you have learned such as the 3Cs, the ABC, or checking out the evidence.)

Coping Cards

- Use coping cards (index cards or business card–size cards) to record your affirmations, things learned. For example, "I don't need to pay attention to my voices." "I can get on with my day and my goals." "Gently turn down the volume." "Think of the voices as background noise." Coaching statements may also be helpful: "You can get through this," "This will pass." (See the list of coping strategies for voices, provided in form 9.8).

Coping Toolkit

• Make a list of the coping strategies you have learned that have been most helpful to you. (Record these on form 4.3, your strengths, coping strategies, and resources list.) Post reminders to yourself on sticky notes and write down reminders on how to do the strategies. Think of cues to remind you to do your coping exercises (when you are at a red light, when you see the color orange, before or after you eat, and so on).

Grounding Exercises

1. Notice yourself in this moment. For example, notice the feel of your butt and back against the chair. Notice the feel of your feet firmly placed on the ground. Notice your hands and arms on the armrest of your chair or feel your arms and hands against your legs. Depending on what works for you, gently place your hand on your chest over your heart area.

2. You may also use stones or other objects to ground you in the present moment. Notice the stones with as many senses as possible.

3. You may also choose to use food items or those with a pleasant odor to engage your senses.

Imagery

• Create an image of a safe, calm, peaceful, or happy place. Use as many of your five senses as possible, including sight, smell, taste, sound, and touch (feel/texture). Guided imagery exercises recorded on a CD, DVD, iPod, or MP3 player can also be used. See our companion website http://www.treatingpsychosis.com for guided imagery exercises.

Learning to Let Go: The Tug of War

• Use a piece of material to have a tug of war. Notice the amount of energy that goes into the struggle. Think about the pros and cons of struggling with distressing voices or thoughts. What would it be like to let the struggle go as much as possible without reacting?

Leaves on a Stream

• Imagine placing thoughts (or voices) on leaves that are gently flowing down a stream and floating out of sight. Other images such as clouds in the sky or a train going by can also let you distance yourself from thoughts or voices.

Progressive Muscle Relaxation

• Tighten and release muscle groups in your body. Start with your feet, then calves, thighs, butt, stomach, chest, arms, hands, neck, and face. Tensing and relaxing muscles helps you let go of the tension you carry in your body. (For a guided exercise, visit our website at http://www.treatingpsychosis.com.)

Thoughts Are Not Facts

- This exercise can be done in session to highlight that thoughts are not facts and to gain distance and perspective around thoughts. Say out loud, "My chair will break in ten seconds," and then notice what happens. Consider what this exercise tells you about your thoughts and how you relate to, or think about, your thoughts. Another thought to check out is *I cannot touch the chair/table/wall*. Say the thought out loud as you put your palm flat on the chair/table/wall. Repeat these thoughts as you touch the chair, table, or wall.

FORM 4.3:   Strengths, Coping Strategies, and Resources List

List your values: _____

List all of your strengths. Add to this list whenever you notice or hear about a new strength, quality, or accomplishment.

1. _____

2. _____

3. _____

4. _____

5. _____

6. _____

7. _____

8. _____

List all of the coping strategies or tools you find helpful. When you find a new coping strategy you like, add it to this list. Keep this list as a reminder of helpful tools you can use to deal with stress and upsetting thoughts or voices.

1. _____

2. _____

3. _____

4. _____

5. _____

6. _____

7. _____

8. _____

Make a list of personal resources or supports you have (for example, health care workers, family, friends, medications, and so on).

1. _____
2. _____
3. _____
4. _____
5. _____
6. _____
7. _____
8. _____

By focusing on positives like the above, we develop strength, resiliency, and the ability to cope with difficulties that can be part of life. By using the list above, you empower yourself and strengthen "positive" or helpful thoughts, feelings, and behaviors in your life.

We all have a tendency to focus on negatives or to look for what might go "wrong." We build our abilities and power by reminding ourselves of strengths, qualities, resources, and coping tools. For more information, see our website (http://www.treatingpsychosis.com) for a list of strengths and virtues.

* Read this list over when you are feeling upset.

* Keep on adding to this list and use it like a toolkit!

FORM 5.1:   **Session Summary**

Session: _____

Date: _____

Topic:_____

Information covered: _____

Coping strategies: _____

Client exercises: _____

What I learned:
(To be filled in collaboratively with clinician in session; e.g., We all have upsetting thoughts; I have the choice about how much time I want to focus on them.)

Between-session practice (homework) for next session:
(To be filled in collaboratively with clinician in session)

Reasons for between-session practice:
(To be filled in collaboratively with clinician in session)

Ideas for troubleshooting barriers to between-session practice:
(To be filled in collaboratively with clinician in session)

Next session

Date: _____ Time: _____

Place: _____

What to bring (e.g., worksheets and handouts):

Questions and/or problems:
(To be filled in by client between sessions)

Things I feel good about; strength(s) and accomplishments:
(To be filled in by client between sessions)

FORM 5.2: Cognitive Behavioral Conceptualization

(Modified with permission from Beck, 1995)

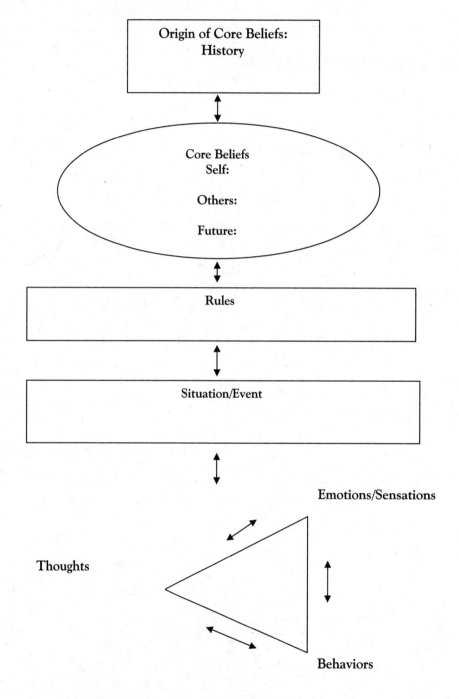

FORM 5.3: **Core Beliefs**

Core beliefs are ideas we have about ourselves and others that can feed into distressing thoughts or unusual beliefs. Core beliefs are beliefs that have been held by a person for a long time that seem true to that person.

Distressing thoughts or voices can reflect core beliefs about oneself, other people, and the future. It is important to think about our core beliefs to develop an accurate and empowering sense of self.

Core beliefs can be healthy or not so healthy. Here are some examples:

- "I am worthwhile" or "I'm not worthwhile."

- "I'm good" or "I'm bad."

- "People are not to be trusted," "People are generally good," or "People are trustworthy."

- "If people really knew me, they would like me" or "If people really knew me, they wouldn't like me."

We tend to focus our attention on things that "fit" with the ideas or beliefs we have about ourselves and others, and we don't pay as much attention to what doesn't "fit." By focusing only on things that fit with our negative, unhealthy, or unhelpful core beliefs, it can feel more and more like a negative belief is true even if it may not be.

Shifting Unhealthy Core Beliefs About Yourself:

Write down any unhealthy or negative core beliefs you have about yourself:

1. _____

2. _____

3. _____

To help make your core beliefs more accurate, write down the following:

- Things I like about myself: _____

- Things others like about me: _____

- Positive things about me are: _____

Try to look for things that don't feed into your negative core beliefs. Over time, try to develop new and healthier core beliefs that fit with your personal values. Write your new core beliefs below. Don't forget to add facts or support for these new core beliefs. Use form 4.3 to remind yourself about your strengths, coping strategies, and resources.

1. _____

2. _____

3. _____

Remember: Shifting core beliefs to be more accurate takes time and effort. But it is worth it! You can start seeing yourself in more healthy and empowering ways.

FORM 5.4:   **Values Worksheet**

Values:

Values are our greatest desires (Harris, 2007). Values are qualities or ways of behaving. They include

- what we want our life to be about;
- what we want to stand for;
- what kind of person we want to be;
- how we want to behave;
- what type of relationships we want to develop; or
- how we want to relate with others and the world.

Values help you work toward the goals that are important to you. Use the Values List on the following page to help you answer the question below, and the questions after that.

1. My personal values or the way I want to be as a person are (for example, *I want to be a caring and compassionate person, I want to be a loving person, I want to be an honest and authentic person*):

Values List: Circle Your Top Five Values

Adaptable	Grateful	Peaceful
Animal lover	Hardworking	Persistent
Appreciative	Health oriented	Respectful
Artistic	Helpful	Responsible
Believe in myself	Honest	Rising above
Calmness	Hopeful	Self-respecting
Caring	Humorous	Sharing
Compassionate	Idealistic	Sociable
Courageous	Insightful	Soulful
Creative	Inspirational	Strong
Dedicated	Joyful	Successful
Determined	Kind	Supportive
Devoted	Leader	Team oriented
Encouraging	Learner	Truthful
Fair	Listener	Trusting
Forgiving	Loving	Understanding
Friendship	Loyal	Visionary
Fun loving	Make a difference	Volunteering
Generous	Motivated	Well-being oriented
Giving back	Patient	Wise

2. Goals linked with value:

3. How important is this value to you on a scale of 1–10 (with 10 being the highest level of importance)?

4. What thoughts, emotions, or symptoms might be barriers to these values and valued goals?

5. How can you motivate yourself to live consistently with these values?

6. How would your life be in one year and in five years from now if you lived consistently with these values?

Please answer the above questions for the following, or complete a values card sort to prioritize values:

- friendship values
- family relationship values
- education and learning values
- work and volunteer values
- health and wellness values
- self-care and personal growth values
- contribution and community values
- meaningful life values
- spiritual and religious values

FORM 5.5: **Goal Setting**

Valued Goals:
A valued goal is a desired outcome. It is something one wishes to do or achieve that has an end point, a finish.

To help you come up with your valued goals, think about the following:

- What is meaningful to me? What would I like my life to be like? What gives me a sense of purpose?
- Where am I going? How am I going to get there?
- What will I be doing when I get there?

Remember to make your valued goals SMART goals. Goals should be specific, measurable, achievable, and time limited (that is, able to be finished).

SMART Goals:

Specific: Is your goal specific enough?

Measurable: How would you know if you completed your goal?

Achievable: Is it possible to do?

Realistic: Can you make it happen?

Time limited: Do you have a date you want finish your goal by?

Please write below your goal(s) for treatment:

1. _____

2. _____

3. _____

Please write below your longer-term goals (personal life and recovery goals):

1. _____

2. _____

3. _____

Remember, when you think of your goals, it can help to think of what you would be doing if you completed your goal. For example, if your goal was to have more friends you would be

- going to activities at the community center and talking to people there;
- going to see a movie with a friend; or
- inviting someone to go for tea.

Think about the steps you would need to do to complete your goal—steps like:

- Talk to people in your group.
- Call an old friend.
- Ask someone you know if they want to go out sometime.
- Go to clubs/activities.

FORM 5.6:   **Treatment Plan**

List strengths, qualities, accomplishments, coping strategies, and resources:

Problem list:

Values:

1. _____

2. _____

3. _____

4. _____

5. _____

Valued goals:
(e.g., less distress around voices in order to do volunteer position one day per week, attend group at community center, and take yoga class, to be compassionate toward myself and others)

Thinking goals:
(e.g., compassionate thinking, helpful thinking that is nonruminative and nonworrying, balanced thinking, constructive thinking, coping thoughts)

Emotional goals:
(e.g., to feel more compassion, grateful, peaceful, happy, content)

Behavioral goals:
(e.g., exercise, developing skills, self-care)

List problems and/or potential barriers to goals:
(e.g., experience, fear and avoidance of voices; suspicions of others, lack of energy, anxiety, and lack of confidence in social situations)

Treatment strategies:
(e.g. mindfulness, voice diary, acceptance of voices, evidence for and against power of voices, behavioral experiments)

FORM 6.1:   Understanding Emotions

(See Leahy, Tirch, and Napolitano, 2011; Linehan, 1993)

Emotions are an important part of being human.

Emotions are temporary—that is, they come and go.

A range of emotions is normal.

Difficult or distressing emotions—such as sadness, anger, fear, and shame—and pleasant emotions—such as happiness, caring, interest, and love—are all normal and a part of life.

Emotions can be helpful. Emotions can alert us to important issues and have a purpose, such as communicating to others, motivating us to act, and validating what we feel.

It can be beneficial to think about our emotions, but the way we think about our emotions can be helpful or unhelpful. For example, we may think an emotion is "unbearable" or "too much to take," or we may think, *I can't handle it*. We can think we shouldn't have a certain kind of emotion. For example, we may think that feeling anger is not okay or that feeling angry says something about who we are.

Trying to stop emotions or avoid emotions can backfire. Instead, it can be helpful to remind yourself that emotions come and go. An image can be helpful, such as thinking of emotions as waves coming and going. Or you can go emotion "surfing," where you ride through the emotions without getting caught in them.

Understanding and accepting a range of emotions, including mixed emotions, can be helpful.

It is possible to increase our experience of positive emotions by noticing and savoring positive emotions and remembering positive memories or experiences.

FORM 6.2:   **Emotion List**

Happy	Proud	Tired
Interested	Excited	Ashamed
Disgusted	Guilty	Loving
Curious	Confident	Loved
Joyful	Surprised	Compassionate
Resentful	Indifferent	Hurt
Optimistic	Relaxed	Regretful
Calm	Grateful	Hopeful
Envious	Jealous	Contemptuous
Empowered	Empowered	Ashamed
Sad	Inspired	Caring
Contented	Anxious	Other:
Safe	Passionate	Other:
Irritated	Angry	Other:

FORM 6.3:   Strategies for Coping with Emotions

Emotions and coping strategies	What is helpful about this strategy?	What is unhelpful about this strategy?	Is there an alternative? What is the most helpful coping strategy?
Emotion: *Anxious* Coping strategies: *Withdraw* *Sleep* *Watch TV*	*I don't notice feeling anxious as much.*	*It keeps me from doing important things in my life.* *I don't get the chance to try other coping strategies.* *I am avoiding.*	1. *Do relaxation exercise, then go out.* 2. *Go for a walk.* 3. *Use my coping cards to talk myself through it.*
Emotions: Coping Strategies:			1. 2. 3.
Emotions: Coping Strategies:			1. 2. 3.
Emotions: Coping Strategies:			1. 2. 3.

(Modified with permission from Morrison et al, 2008)

FORM 6.4: Valued Activities, Willingness, Values, and Goals

When it feels difficult or stressful to do something, it can be hard to motivate ourselves to do what it takes to work toward our goals. At these times, it can be helpful to remind ourselves of what is important to us, including our values and meaningful goals.

Instructions: Notice the activities that are hard for you to do in working toward your goals. In column 1, write the activities you need to do to work toward your goals. In column 2, write reminders that will help you be more willing or motivated to do these activities. In columns 3 and 4, list the values that you will base your goal(s) on and the goal(s) you are working toward. Once you have completed this form, read it again to motivate yourself.

Activities (the steps to take to work toward goals)	Willingness Motivators (reminders that help me to do what it takes to live by my values and work toward my goals)	Values	Goals
Examples: *Get out of bed* *Get dressed* *Take the bus*	Examples: *It is more important to work on my goals than to avoid feelings.* *I can do this even if it is hard.* *I am willing to feel some anxiety to work toward my goals.* *No pain, no gain.* *Go in the direction of your dreams, not your fears.*	Examples: *Being kind to others*	Examples: *Volunteering to help others*

FORM 6.5:   Compassion-Focused Exercises

(See Germer, 2009; Gilbert, 2009; Gilbert & Choden, 2013; Neff, 2011; Tirch, 2012; and our website http://www.treatingpsychosis.com for more examples of compassion-focused exercises.)

In CFT, we develop warmth and soothing toward ourselves and others. For many, this can be very difficult to do at first. Talk with your clinician and go at a pace that is right for you. It is important to gradually try these exercises and make them a part of your everyday life and way of being. This takes courage, practice, and time. It can be hard to feel positive emotions, soothing, and self-compassion. If it is difficult for you, it can be helpful to start with exercises for developing caring and compassion toward others first. But remember: your compassion is not complete if it does not include *you*! Below we describe a number of compassion-focused skill development exercises you can do to develop and enhance your care and compassion toward yourself and others.

Compassionate Self Exercise

A good place to begin with compassion-focused experiences is this Compassionate Self exercise. Begin by grounding your body and doing belly breathing as described in the coping exercises (form 4.2). It can be helpful to place your hand over your heart and to do a very gentle half-smile. In addition, try to imagine yourself becoming a compassionate and wise being. It may be helpful to think of yourself at your best—those times when you have been kind and caring.

Try to practice each day in different ways and at different times, such as before you get out of bed, when having a bath, while on the bus, while waiting for an appointment, and so on. Put reminders about your compassionate self on a coping card. Remember to bring compassion to your compassion-focused exercises. Set the intention to practice and compassionately encourage your practice.

Compassionate Attention

- I will pay attention, in the present moment, in a caring way.
- I will focus on compassionate mindfulness.
- If I notice myself ruminating, I will refocus my attention through mindfulness or focusing on my strengths and my goals.
- I will focus on things that are helpful to myself and others.
- I will focus on what is supportive.
- I will pay attention to my "wise" mind and to the wisom I have generated.
- I will notice when I am worrying and bring my attention back to the moment.
- I will use mindfulness to guide my attention to caring and compassion.

Compassionate Behavior

- I will talk to someone I trust and get the support and understanding I need.

- I will do self-care and pamper myself when I am going through a tough time.

- I will go at a pace that is good for me. No pressure. I will just gently move toward what is important to me.

- I will try to give people the benefit of the doubt and see if there is anything I can do to help.

- I will try smiling at others.

- I will help others out.

- I will do random acts of kindness!

- I will say kind things, not hurtful things.

- I will be mindful or imagine compassion flowing out to others.

- I will do mindfulness to bring compassion and caring to myself.

Compassionate Thinking and Reasoning

- I am okay. By being understanding and caring with myself, I can work toward my values and goals.

- I did not ask for the psychosis or my busy, tricky brain, but I can choose to take care of myself just like I would someone else.

- I am not alone. Other people have difficulties like this. I can be gentle with myself rather than judging or criticizing myself.

- I can do it. Through soothing and caring, I can get through.

- This feeling will not last. I've gotten through it before and I will again. Breathe!

- Instead of being self-critical, I can focus on my strengths and accomplishments.

- Instead of thinking about myself with judgment and criticism, I can be gently self-correcting in my thinking and learn from the experience.

- Instead of thinking about something over and over again in a judging or self-critical way (ruminating), I can refocus my thinking on caring, problem solving, or coping.

- I will reason through hurtful thinking by gently checking it out, examining the evidence, thinking about more helpful ways of understanding the situation, and so on.

- I will use the 4Cs—catch it, check it, and change it with compassion—for my thinking when it is not helpful.

- I will try to understand what it is like for others. They are probably dealing with tough stuff, too.
- I will try to think about putting myself in other people's shoes.

Compassionate Emotions and Sensory Feelings

- I will try to generate feelings of caring.
- I will create soothing feelings.
- I will remember what it felt like when I felt soothed and cared for.
- To enhance nurturing or positive emotions, I will use another 3Cs. The 3Cs are used to (1) compassionately catch or create the positive emotion, moment, or memory, (2) consolidate the emotion through savoring it, and then (3) connect the memory and emotion to neutral or distressing experiences to gently soften them.
- I will try using kindness to others so they can feel my caring.
- I will be understanding and supportive of others so they can feel cared for.

Compassionate Imagery/Fantasy

- Develop an image of my compassionate self using all my senses. I will use this compassionate self-image to help me when I notice I am worrying or ruminating.
- Develop an image of an extremely kind and compassionate being or object, such as an animal, plant, person, ideal, or something else.
- Use guided imagery to create a safe place.
- Imagine a compassionate color—that is, a color that is linked with a feeling of calmness and kindness.

Compassionate Motivation

- I will focus on the intention to be caring and compassionate.
- My intention will be to live my values of kindness and compassion.
- I intend to bring kindness to myself and to what I do.
- My intention is to be compassionate toward others in life. Life can be hard for all of us.

FORM 6.6:   Thinking Styles

Not all thoughts we have are accurate or helpful. Noticing or "catching" your thoughts and "checking" thoughts out can be helpful. Identifying and understanding your thinking styles can help you to consider different ways of thinking about yourself, others, or the future. Typical thinking styles or "traps" are listed below. Use this list (Beck et al., 2009) to notice or "catch" unhelpful thinking styles and shift to more helpful thinking styles.

Zebra Thinking or Black-and-White Thinking
You see things as black or white. You say things are "good" or "bad" but see nothing in between.

> *Example:* Because you have an illness you tell yourself, *I'm a failure.*

Labeling
You label yourself or others instead of using less extreme ways of thinking about behaviors or events.

> *Example:* "I'm a loser." "He's evil."

Overgeneralization
You come to negative conclusions that spread to more than the situation.

> *Example:* Because someone didn't want to go for a coffee with you, you think, *No one likes me.*

Elephant Thinking or Catastrophizing (also called fortune telling)
You think the worst will happen or make HUGE problems out of small problems.

> *Example:* "I'll never be able to do anything."

Frog Thinking or Jumping to Conclusions
You "jump to a conclusion" without thinking about other possibilities.

> *Example:* When people are laughing, you think they are laughing at you without checking out other explanations.

Skunk Thinking, Stinking Thinking (also called "emotional reasoning")
You think something is true because you "feel" like it is true.

> *Example:* "I feel like he is watching me." (You believe it is true even though the facts show it isn't.)

Magnification

When you evaluate yourself, another person, or a situation, you magnify the positive (or the negative).

Example: "He always does everything perfectly. I could never do that."

Dismissing the Positive

You reject or don't believe good things about yourself.

Example: "She is just saying that to make me feel better."

Mental Filter

You pay attention to one negative detail and don't notice the rest—like all the things you do well.

Example: You make a mistake on your homework—"I can't do anything right."

Mind Reading

You believe you know what others are thinking and don't think about other possibilities.

Example: "They think I'm crazy."

Personalization (the focus is on you like a spotlight)

You believe others are behaving negatively because of you, without thinking of other explanations.

Example: (when others are laughing at a joke) "Those people are laughing at me."

Blame

You believe others have negative or hurtful plans or are at fault.

Example: "They will reject me because they think I have a mental illness."

"Should" and "Must" Statements

You have a fixed idea of how you or others should behave, think, or feel.

Examples: "I should never make a mistake." "I must do what my voices say."

All of us can jump to conclusions at times. Sometimes we can believe that we or others have special/supernatural powers and abilities without checking this out to see if it is factual. Sometimes we can think that people's facial expressions are angry or mean when they are not feeling that way.

Toolkit for Unhelpful Thinking Styles

Cognitive flexibility: Be flexible in your thinking. Consider more helpful explanations.

Metathinking: Think about your thinking. Is it helpful?

Decentering: Take the focus off yourself—make sure you are not thinking that the spotlight is on you.

Activity: Do meaningful activities. Work toward your goals. Don't get caught in unhelpful thinking.

Examine the evidence: Check out the evidence for and against your thoughts to see how helpful and accurate your thinking is.

Do self-coaching: Talk yourself through it and tell yourself you can do it.

Read a coping card: Read a card that has a strength or coping information written on it.

Write out the pros and cons of thinking this way: Think about the benefits and drawbacks of thinking this way, and think in ways that are the most workable.

Do what is helpful.

Decatastrophize: Don't always think about the worst.

Find the lesson: Try to learn something from the situation instead of going over and over it in your head.

Think of alternative explanations: Think about other ways of thinking about situations.

Think about blame: Are you laying too much blame on one person?

Do an experiment: Check it out. Test it out.

Ask: Is this a fact or a thought?

Ask: What would someone else think?

Ask: How would you think about this a year from now?

Use the court of law approach: Pretend you are thinking about this like a lawyer. Think about the facts and the evidence.

Give the person the benefit of the doubt.

Don't jump to conclusions without proof.

Engage in factual reasoning, not emotional reasoning: Think about things based on the facts, not on how you feel.

Think of the best possible outcome.

Brainstorm other ways of thinking about the situation.

Ask trusted others what they think.

Postpone your conclusion: Don't just jump to a conclusion. Think about it for a while.

Try thinking more hopefully.

Think of it from the other person's point of view.

Seek first to understand before assuming.

Cope, don't catastrophize.

Think of other explanations.

Look at the big picture: Put things in perspective.

Think about it from different vantage points, views, or perspectives.

Think about what others would say.

Think about how things could go right.

Be your own best friend.

Practice compassion with your inner critic or inner bully.

Look for things that don't make sense or fit with your thinking.

Notice errors in your thinking.

Use your logical mind, not your emotional mind.

Label actions, not people: For example, the behavior is hurtful, not the whole person.

Think of what you would *prefer* to do instead of using harsher terms for alternatives like "I should" or "I must."

Ask others what they think: Take a survey!

FORM 6.7: The 3Cs and 4Cs—Catch It, Check It, Change It (with Compassion)

Catch It (or notice it)	Check It	Change It	Change It with Compassion (see Change It section as well)
Catch or notice the distressing thought or image.	Check out the evidence for and against the thought. Ask yourself, What would a friend, family member, or health care provider say? Ask yourself, Is this a helpful way to think about it? Ask yourself, Is my thought based on facts or just feelings? Ask yourself, Am I thinking about the worst thing? Ask yourself, What would I say to a friend?	It's just a thought. Give others the benefit of the doubt. See it through compassionate eyes to find a coping response or a caring way of thinking. Come up with a more reasonable, helpful, or rational thought. Change your thought to one that is based on checking out the facts.	See and think about the situation through compassionate eyes. Think of the situation with more self-compassion and kindness. Think of the situation and others in a more compassionate, understanding way.

FORM 6.8: Positive Emotion Exercises

Use your five senses (seeing, hearing, smelling, touching, and tasting) to generate positive images.

Use the five senses to remember positive memories.

Count and let go of self-judgments.

Nourish your spirit.

Savor experiences.

Notice positive emotions. Savor positive emotions and gently let feelings come and go.

Create positive emotions by focusing on something pleasant.

Enjoy, linger, soak in, and hold on to positive feelings.

Savor personal strengths or qualities.

Appreciate three things before going to sleep.

List three good things in life.

List three things each day that you are grateful for.

List your top five strengths.

Do a gratitude practice: write a letter to thank someone.

Allow thoughts to come and go.

Develop empathy and self-compassion.

Label emotions with gentleness—this calms the brain. When you name it, you tame it.

Soften, soothe, allow.

Be mindful, grateful, playful.

FORM 7.1:   ABC for Action

Fill out the form below when you are thinking about doing an activity.

1. Write down the activity under the Activity column.

2. Write down your inaction and action thoughts and beliefs.

3. Write down the consequences: your emotions and behaviors during and after you did or did not do the activity.

Activity (the activity you want to do)	Beliefs/Thoughts/Images (about doing the activity)	Consequences (emotional and behavioral)
Inaction Belief (Examples: "I'm too tired." "It won't be any fun." "I won't be able to do it.")		
Activity:	My beliefs, thoughts, or images about doing the activity:	Emotions (How did I feel after I did not do the activity?): Behaviors (What did I do during and after when I would have done the activity?):
Action Belief (Examples: "I get more energy when I get going." "It may be better than I think it will be." "I'll do my best—that's what counts.")		
Activity (same as above):	My beliefs, thoughts, or images about doing the activity:	Emotions (How did I feel after I did the activity?): Behaviors (What did I do when I did the activity and after?):

Form 7.2: Activity Form

(Modified with permission from Lejuez et al., 2001)

Instructions: Complete the form below by writing down the activities you did (or plan to do) in each day and time slot. You may also write down the emotion you felt when doing the activity—using a scale of 0–10, with 10 being the highest level of the emotion (for example, E=5, for the emotion "happy")—and the difficulty of the activity, using the same scale with 10 being the highest level of difficulty (for example, D=6).

	Mon	Tues	Wed	Thurs	Fri	Sat	Sun
7–9 a.m.	*Ex.* Got out of bed: E = 5 D = 6						
9–11 a.m.							
11–1 p.m.							
1–3 p.m.							
3–5 p.m.							
5–7 p.m.							
7–9 p.m.							
9–11 p.m.							
11–7 a.m.							

FORM 7.3:   Values and Valued Activities

Please write down your personal values, and the valued activities that will help you to live a life consistent with those values as well as work toward your valued goals.

Values	Valued Activities	Valued Goals

FORM 7.4:   **Emotion and Mastery Form**

Week of _____ to _____

Use the table that follows to complete this activity. (1) List the activities you plan to do. (2) Write down how long you plan to spend on the activity or the time at which you plan to do the activity. (3) Write down the emotion that you expect to feel while doing the activity; rate how much of the emotion you expect to feel with 10 being the highest level of the emotion. (4) Now rate how difficult you think it will be to do the activity (0 for no difficulty to 10 for most difficulty).

(5) When you've completed the activity, note this in the fifth column. (6) Then rerate the actual emotion you felt when you did the activity and (7) the level of difficulty you had doing the activity. Were your expectations accurate? Did it go as you planned? What did you learn?

To start, write down a goal, value, or theme for the week's activities to help remind you of your overall aims.

Goal/Value/Theme for Week:_____

Activity	Amount/Time (Planned)	Expected Emotion (1–10)	Expected Difficulty (0–10)	Amount/Time (Actual)	Actual Emotion (1–10)	Actual Difficulty (0–10)

FORM 7.5: **Activity Ladder**

With your clinician, list the activities you think would be helpful in working toward your valued goals. Estimate how difficult you expect the activity would be using the scale below. Keep in mind how much you avoid the activity, and how much effort you think you would need to complete it.

0	25	50	75	100
No avoidance	Little avoidance	Usually avoided	Avoided as a rule	Total avoidance
or	*or*	*or*	*or*	*or*
Effortless	Needs some effort	Requires great effort	Takes extreme effort	Seems impossible

Key Value(s): _____

Key Goal(s): _____

Item	Activity	Difficulty (0–10)
1		
2		
3		
4		
5		
6		
7		
8		
9		
10		
11		
12		
13		
14		
15		

FORM 8.1:   Working with Paranoid Thoughts

(For clinicians.)

1. Go from *abstract to concrete*. For example, "You say you're a robot; what do you mean by a 'robot'?" (It's important to extract as much detail as possible.)

2. Use plenty of *reflection*, repeating back what you've heard. Not only does it help engagement by letting clients know you've heard and understood what they've said, it also gives you time to think about what you're doing!

3. What is the *evidence* for clients believing what they do? For example, "What makes you think that?"

4. Is there anything that makes them think that they might have *jumped to a conclusion* or gotten it wrong?

5. *Consider alternative explanations.* Is there any other way of seeing things or of understanding the evidence? For example, "You say that you think that every time someone touches his or her nose it's a code saying they think you're gay. Could there be any other explanation for why some people touch their noses?"

6. If the person cannot come up with any alternative ways of seeing the situation, then you may have to generate alternatives. For example, "You have told me that there is a UFO hovering over your house every night. I know this sounds crazy, but could it be a recurring vivid nightmare or a burglar light or some other local phenomenon?"

7. Use *behavioral experiments* to test out beliefs *and* alternative beliefs.

Remember: Clients should do the thinking...*you're just there to facilitate*!

Keep in mind that people with delusions:

- tend to jump to conclusions (use less information before they make up their minds), so we are guiding them to consider other elements of evidence.

- do not tend to look for disconfirmatory evidence.

- are less likely to have alternative explanations available to them.

FORM 8.2:   Pie Chart for Alternative Explanations

(Modified with permission from Leahy, 2003)

Thought:

Rationally how much do you believe this? _____% (0–100%)

Emotionally how much do you believe this? _____% (0–100%)

What other reasons might there be for this?

1. _____

2. _____

3. _____

4. _____

5. _____

6. _____

7. _____

This circle represents the "reasons pie." We can split this pie into slices, with each slice representing how much another reason might have contributed to an event (bigger slice = more responsible). If we add up every reason's "slice" of pie, this should add up to 100 percent responsibility, as every reason played a role in the event happening. Using the list you've generated above, starting at the bottom of the list, give each reason a "slice" of the pie, representing how responsible it is for what happened. After you've finished this, the "slice" that is left over is how much the initial reason you gave is considered to be responsible for what happened.

Rerate your belief in the original reason you thought of (0–100%): _____%

Rerate how much you think other reasons contribute to the event (0–100%): _____%

Alternative thought, if you can come up with a more reasonable thought:

_____

FORM 8.3: Behavioral Experiments for Distressing Voices, Thoughts, or Delusions

(Modified with permission from Morrison et al., 2008)

Thought/Belief to be tested:

Possible alternative thoughts/beliefs:

Anxiety level predicted: _____ %

Belief in the thought (0–100) before behavioral experiment: _____%

Belief (0–100) after experiment: _____%

Experiment to test belief:	Predicted outcome:	Safety behaviors to be dropped:	Coping strategies:	What did we find out?	What is the best explanation? Give % belief scores.

We always need at least two experiments. The first of these is done with support in a nonchallenging environment.

FORM 9.1: Voice Diary

(Inspired by Turkington et al., 2009)

Just as you might write down thoughts on a thought record or thought diary, writing down information about your voices can be helpful. First, try writing down the situation or event that was happening when you heard the voice (column 1), then write down word for word exactly what the voice said (column 2). Try to see what you can learn about your voices. Do you notice any patterns? When do you tend to hear your voices? What do your voices tend to say? When you are ready, do columns 3, 4, 5, and 6. Rate the distress you feel (0–100, with 100 representing the most distress) when you hear your voices (column 3), and what emotions you feel—for example, fear, anger, sadness, shame, or happiness (column 4). List the coping strategies you use (column 5), and rate your distress after you use the coping strategy (column 6). By learning more about your voices, you can empower yourself and spend more of your time and energy working toward your goals.

1. Situation, Event, Activity, Unpleasant Physiological Reaction	2. Voice (Who? Origin? Content of voice?)	3. Rate Distress of Voice (0–100)	4. Emotion(s)	5. Coping Strategies (List and describe)	6. Outcome: Rate Distress of Voice (0–100)

FORM 9.2: Cognitive Behavioral Conceptualization for Voices

(Modified with permission from Beck, 1995)

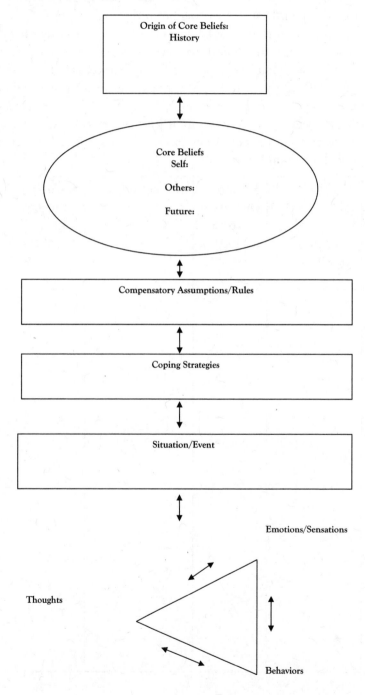

FORM 9.3:   ABC for Voices

Instructions:

1. In the first column, write down what the voice said.

2. In the second column under the "distressing belief," write your beliefs, thoughts, or images about what the voice said. Think of an alternative, more helpful belief, thought, or image about the voice, and write this under column 2 for the "helpful belief example."

3. Write down your emotions and behaviors for the distressing belief and the helpful belief.

4. Notice if there is a difference in your emotions and behaviors in the distressing belief and helpful belief examples.

1. Activating Event = Voice (same in both examples)	2. Beliefs/Thoughts/Images About Voices	3. Consequences (emotions and behaviors)
Distressing Belief:		
		Emotions: Behaviors:
Helpful/Alternative Belief:		
		Emotions: Behaviors:

FORM 9.4:   Pros and Cons of Beliefs About the Content of Voices

Describe what the voice says:	
Describe your belief about what the voice says:	
List pros/advantages of believing the voice:	List cons/disadvantages of believing the voice:
List alternative understandings or explanations:	

FORM 9.5: Evidence for and Against Beliefs About the Content of Voices

(Modified with permission from Morrison et al., 2008)

Belief about voice content: _____

_____

_____

_____

Rate belief conviction (0–100%): _____

Rate distress associated with this belief: (0–100%): _____

Evidence for the belief: _____ | Evidence against the belief: _____

_____ | _____

_____ | _____

_____ | _____

List other possible beliefs about the content of the voice: _____

_____

_____

_____

FORM 9.6: Evidence for and Against Beliefs About the Cause or Origin of Voices

(Modified with permission from Morrison et al., 2008)

Belief about the cause of my voices: _____

_____

_____

_____

Rate belief conviction (0–100%): _____

Rate distress associated with this belief: (0–100%): _____

Evidence for the belief: _____	Evidence against the belief: _____
_____	_____
_____	_____
_____	_____

List other possible beliefs about the cause of your voices: _____

_____

_____

_____

FORM 9.7: Pie Chart for Explanation of Voices

(Modified with permission from Leahy, 2003)

Consider the different pieces in the "pie" below. Each piece represents a possible explanation for the cause of the voices.

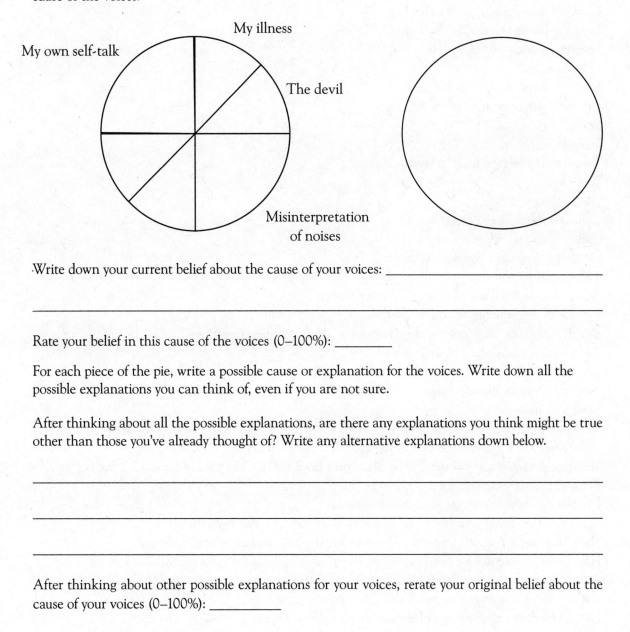

Write down your current belief about the cause of your voices: _____

_____

Rate your belief in this cause of the voices (0–100%): _____

For each piece of the pie, write a possible cause or explanation for the voices. Write down all the possible explanations you can think of, even if you are not sure.

After thinking about all the possible explanations, are there any explanations you think might be true other than those you've already thought of? Write any alternative explanations down below.

_____

_____

_____

After thinking about other possible explanations for your voices, rerate your original belief about the cause of your voices (0–100%): _____

FORM 9.8: Coping Strategies for Voices

Thoughts or Actions
Hum.
Talk silently to yourself.
Count or sing under your breath.
Say to yourself, "This will pass."
Listen to music.
Play the guitar.
Meditate or pray.
Use a mantra or positive self-statement.
Paint.
Use a peaceful image.
Take a warm bath, or walk in the fresh air.
Work out.
Use a relaxation tape.
Call your therapist or caregiver.
Call or visit a friend.
Go to the drop-in or community center.
Try something new.
Watch TV, or listen to the radio, a CD, or your iPod.
Go on the computer or YouTube.
Watch a YouTube TED talk on the computer—hear something inspiring.
Read a magazine, poetry, or short story.
Read a self-help book.
Work on a puzzle, like a crossword or Sudoku.
Take your meds.
Correct errors in your thinking about the voices. For example, "The voices do not always stop me."
Think logically about the voices. For example, "I am a good person."
Tell the voices that you will think about them only from 5:00 to 5:30 p.m., or some other time of the day.
Remember that you don't need to obey the voices.
Dismiss the voices, or teach the voices manners.
Remind yourself that your voices are just sounds; no one else can hear them.
Show that you can control the voices by bringing them on and switching them off.
Have a ten-minute slot for thinking happy thoughts at a particular time each day.
Remember voices are common: "This happens to lots of people, like Anthony Hopkins."
Use calm thinking to reduce angry thoughts about voices.
List the evidence against the unhelpful thoughts about voices.

Practice coping with your voices in your imagination.

Use imagery to practice coping with the voices differently.

Role-play for and against the voices.

Put the voices in the witness box.

Use a diary to plan your time and daily activities so that voices don't distract you or stress you out.

Use a voice diary in a scientific manner to check out patterns and themes.

Use mindfulness, let the voice come and go and don't get caught up in it.

Think about the big picture—put thinking about voices in perspective.

Do things to increase your self-esteem.

Change negative thoughts about yourself to more accurate thoughts.

Think about your thinking about your voices. Use helpful ways of thinking about your voices.

Accept the voices and let them go.

Be assertive with your voices.

Teach your voices limits or boundaries.

Remind yourself that voices are just part of an illness.

Think of people who have coped with voices.

Think about cultural understandings—in some cultures, voices are a gift.

Use a diary to write down things you feel good about—like friendships, or pleasant experiences you've had.

Remind yourself that you have coped with the voices before and you will do it again.

Prove with your actions that the voices are inaccurate—that you're not what they say you are.

Be extra kind to yourself.

Be your own best friend.

Values

Connect with your personal values to help you work toward your goals rather than struggling with your voices.

Consider whether one of your values is compassion and caring for yourself when you hear your voices.

What sort of person do you want to be? Do you want to be kind with yourself?

Do what you want to stand for and ignore the voices.

Think about your purpose and do it.

Do what is meaningful. Don't get distracted by your voices.

Respect and motivate yourself to move toward your goals, not your voices.

Notice your voices and don't get caught up in them.

Do activities to move toward your goals.

Do effective action—do what is helpful.

Do what works.

Move in the direction of your hopes, not your fears.

Compassion

Change your relationship with the voices.

Use compassionate intention. Focus your intentions on kindness.

Use compassionate attention. Focus on kindness and caring.

Think compassionate thoughts about yourself.

Think compassionately about others.

Act or behave compassionately toward yourself.

Be kind and caring with yourself.

Speak compassionately.

Talk to yourself compassionately.

Think of a compassionate image—for example, nature, an animal, a person, or a special being.

Cherish a compassionate memory.

Reflect on compassionate role models—the Dalai Lama or Mother Teresa or a caregiver, health care provider, therapist, family, member, friend, or others.

Make compassionate coping cards.

Write a compassionate letter to yourself.

Nourish compassion—water it, feed it.

Mindfulness Approaches

Use mindfulness bells. Have a reminder that brings you back to the present moment.

Breathe mindfully.

Eat and taste mindfully.

Walk mindfully.

Listen mindfully.

Smell mindfully. Smell the roses!

Touch mindfully.

Be mindfully aware of what you see.

Sit mindfully.

Use a coping card to remind you to focus on the breath or use mindfulness.

Think of what you are grateful for.

Think of a positive memory.

Notice distress you hold on to and begin to let go or forgive.

Savor positive or pleasant experiences.

Use a peaceful-place image.

Connect with the Present Moment

Use mindfulness—learn to focus on bringing it into your daily life.

Awareness: notice what is around (other than voices).

Use your five senses to notice other things and to ground yourself in the here and now.

Notice what you smell.

Notice what you touch.

Notice what you see— the sky, the picture on the wall, your shirt, and so on.

Notice what you hear—other than or in addition to your voices.

Notice what you taste— food, drink, and so on.

Use Imagery for the Fleeting Nature of Voices

Leaves on a stream: imagine putting your voices on leaves on a stream and watching them float out of sight.

Imagine your voices as clouds in the sky.

Your voices are waves—you're not caught up in them.

Your voices are writings in the sand—they wash away with no lasting effect.

Your voices are a noisy bus passenger that you do not need to focus on.

Hearing your voices is like whitewater rafting—you ride through the tough stuff.

Voice surfing.

Use Imagery to Have an Effect on the Voices

Throw a blanket over the voices.

Turn the volume down on the voices: imagine a dial or knob like a radio to turn the volume down.

Use the image of an on/off knob or button to turn the voices off.

Gain Distance and Perspective from Your Thoughts About Your Voices

Relate to thoughts about your voices in new and different ways.

Let go of self-bullying.

Let go of self-limiting thoughts and beliefs.

Remember thoughts are thoughts, not facts.

Thoughts about voices may or may not be true.

Remember voices are just sounds, words, stories, or pieces of language.

Thoughts about voices may or may not be helpful: pay attention to those that are helpful in moving you toward your values and goals.

Thoughts about voices and voices themselves may or may not be wise. Therefore, decide if you should follow their advice.

Thoughts are not threats.

Thoughts about voices may or may not be important.

Remember that voices are just a string of words.

Remember that voices may not be wise; you do not have to obey them.

Say, "I'm having the thought that my voices are too much to bear, but I can get through this."

Say. "I notice I'm having the thought that the voice is…" (completing the statement as appropriate).

Acceptance

Let go of struggling with voices.

Make room for unpleasant as well as pleasant reality.

I'm not keen on hearing the voices, but I can cope with them.

I don't like having voices, but I can accept they are part of my illness and carry on.

I may feel or think certain ways when I hear the voices, but I can keep on going.

A—accept thoughts, feelings, experiences. C—connect with my values. T—take effective action (Harris, 2007).

Think of ways to stop struggle, avoidance, and loss of the moment.

Use music or other sounds.

Remember your mind is a fabulous storyteller—you can handle your mind's stories about your voices.

Think of voices as background noise.

Metathinking: think about the way you think about your voices; does it make sense?

Question the evidence for your voices and against your voices.

Question your thoughts about your voices.

Just because you hear voices, does it mean what the voices say is true?

Look for proof.

Consider other explanations for voices.

Consider how helpful it is to spend so much time thinking about your voices.

Do what helps.

Do what is workable.

Remember not to think the worst.

Remember not to catastrophize.

Think of what you can learn from how you deal with your voices.

Brainstorm different ways to deal with voices.

Distribute responsibility fairly.

Practice or role-play how you want to handle voices.

Check out your voices: do an experiment to test them out.

Tape your voices: what do you hear?

Engage in positive memory attention training.

Increase your sense of control by reminding yourself about times and places where voices are less common.

Discuss the beliefs you have about your voices.

Think, *How can I help myself? Are there any benefits to holding on to my voices or beliefs about voices that get in the way of me letting them go?*

Use helpful self-talk for the voices.

Self-coach and talk yourself through it: with practice it will become easier.

Shift your thinking: focus on something else that is helpful or productive.

Do something else.

Use a signal or cue to remind yourself to shift from focusing on voices.

Distract yourself with something else.

Remember that you don't have to pay attention to everything you hear (like background TV, radio).

Pay attention to other noises and sounds.

Notice negative thinking about voices.

Notice thinking traps about voices.

Reduce triggers for voices. (Be careful of safety behaviors or using avoidance of voices in a way that indicates to you that you can't handle the voices.) Remember that you can cope with your voices, but you may decide you want to reduce triggers for voices in some situations.

Avoid scary movies, if they make the voices worse.

Avoid angry music.

Avoid spy or crime novels.

More Thinking Strategies

Think, *What can I do to cope?*

Think, *What can I do to make the voices better?*

What would a friend say?

What would a caregiver or health care provider say?

Have a voice buddy or voice coach.

Use what has worked for you in the past to deal with your voices.

Ask yourself these questions (see Harris, 2009):

- Is this a familiar thought or voice?
- Have I heard this thought or voice before?
- Is there anything to be gained by listening to this thought or voice again?
- Does listening to my voices or believing my voices
  - help me to live the kind of life I want to live?
  - help me create the types of relationships I want to have?
  - help me be in touch with what I really value?
  - help me to be the kind of person I want to be?
  - help me to work toward and create a full and meaningful life?
  - help me make the most out of my life?

Don't take the voices too seriously.

Are the voices telling me a familiar story—for example, the "I'm not good enough story"?

Name the story and decide if this is the story you want to continue to pay attention to and believe.

Use the silly voices technique: say what your voice says in a silly way (for example, as Donald Duck).

Repeat what your voice says over and over fast.

The voice says, "You are a bad person," and you say, "You are a banana."

Thank the voices: "Thanks for coming by—catch you later."

Do pleasurable things.

Say the serenity prayer.

Accept those problems that can't be solved.

Make peace with voices.

Let go of the battle with the voices.

Notice how you relate to your voices.

Notice how you react to your voices.

Think of voices like a TV or CD playing in the background.

Notice when the voice hooks you and carries you away.

Unhook yourself from your voices.

Assume good intentions of others.

Assume the voices have it wrong.

Focus on the good stuff in life—what you have done, not what you haven't done.

Do self-care.

Pamper yourself.

Play with a pet.

Think of your accomplishments.

Make plans for the future.

Keep focused on your goals.

Think what would you do if the voices were not around and do it.

Do what interests you (or interested you) whether the voices are there or not.

Like a time machine, think about the voices like they happened a long time ago.

Notice and name five things around you.

Notice what you see and feel.

Think, *What would I do differently if the voices weren't here?*—and do it!

Think, *What would my life be like if I didn't pay as much attention to the voices?*—and make it happen!

Breathe. Your breath can be like an anchor in crashing waves: it may not stop the waves, but it can help steady you.

Think, *I may not be able to stop the waves, but I can take up voice surfing.*

Do what you want to do in spite of the voices.

Live a full and meaningful life!

FORM 9.9: Behavioral Experiment for Beliefs about Voices

(Modified with permission from Morrison et al., 2008)

Belief about voice to be tested: (For example, "The voices are all-powerful and will hurt me if I don't do what they say.")

_____

_____

Belief (0–100%):

Belief before experiment: _____100_____ %

Belief after experiment: _____80_____ %

Experiment to Test Belief	Likely Problems	Strategies to Deal with Problems	Expected Outcome	Actual Outcome	Alternative Belief
Refuse to carry out command of voices to hurt myself by stabbing myself in the arm with pen.	*Inconclusive: Gently poking self with pen (doing appeasement behaviors).*	*Try with and without poking myself with a pen (doing it without the appeasement behavior).*	*The voices will hurt me.*	*The voices did not hurt me.*	*If I disobey the voices, they don't (always) hurt me. Maybe I am giving them too much power.*

FORM 9.10: Voice Avoidance Hierarchy

List of situations with voices avoided due to fear/anxiety about the voice (If there is more than one voice, start with the least distressing voice first.)	Anxiety (0–100%)	Avoidance (0–100% of time)
Thinking about the voice		
Talking about the voice		
Writing about the voice		
Listening to the voice		
Imagining the voice		
Talking about the voice with a friend		
Talking about the voice with a family member		
Talking about the voice with a health care provider		
Bringing the voice on in session with a health care provider		
Bringing the voice on outside of session with a health care provider		
Bringing the voice on with a safe other		
Bringing the voice on by self at home		
Bringing the voice on by self away from home		
Clinician role-playing the voice and me responding		
Role-playing the voice and pretending that a friend hears the voice		
Role-playing the voice with clinician responding		
Clinician role-playing voice and me responding		
Two-chair exercise responding to voice		
Coping with the voice outside of session		
Not responding to commands of the voice but doing something to appease the voice, or make it happy even though I didn't do what it said		
Not responding to commands of the voice		
Other, please list:		
Other, please list:		
Other, please list:		

Voice Avoidance Hierarchy for Situations

List of situations avoided due to fear or anxiety regarding voices	Situation Avoided? Yes/No	Not Avoided but Causes Anxiety? Yes/No
Travel by bus or train		
Listening to the radio		
Watching TV		
Being at home		
Leaving home		
Gym		
Community center		
Groups		
Classrooms		
Theaters/movies		
Shopping malls		
Church/spiritual center		
Hospital or medical clinic		
Restaurants		
Dentist		
Doctor		
Parties		
Being with unfamiliar people I don't know		
Being with people I know		
Auditoriums		
Cars		
Other, please list:		
Other, please list:		
Other, please list:		
Other, please list:		

FORM 9.11:   Pros and Cons of Time Focused on Voices

What are my values? What are my goals?	
Describe time focused on voices (e.g., listening to voices, talking to voices, watching out for triggers for voices, avoiding voices, etc.)	
How much time do I spend on my voices per week?	
How much time do I spend on my voices per day?	
Pros or advantages of spending time focused on the voices:	Cons or disadvantages of spending time focused on the voices:
What would I rather be spending my time doing?	

FORM 9.12:   Action Plan for Voices

Sometimes voices or upsetting thoughts can get in the way of values and goals. Planning for challenges to working toward your goals can help.

1. Remind yourself of your values—these can keep you on track each and every day.

    My values:

    _____

    _____

2. Think about your valued activities or things you want to do to work toward your goals.

    My valued activities (things that are helpful to do each day):

    _____

    _____

    Things that I can do each day to work toward value-based living and goals:

    _____

    _____

3. Problem-solve possible challenges to working toward your goals. Here are some examples of possible challenges to working toward goals:
    *   avoiding doing what is important because of my voices
    *   believing the voices instead of working toward my goals
    *   struggling with my voices or wasting time on my voices instead of working on my goals

    My challenges:

    _____

    _____

    Ways to overcome challenges (for example, ignore my voices and do it anyway, book voice time for later in the day so I have time to work on my goals, or do a self-compassion imagery exercise):

    _____

    _____

See the Coping Strategies for Voices (form 9.8) for more ideas.

FORM 10.1:   Staying Well Plan

Being healthy and staying well is important for all of us. It can be very helpful to come up with a staying well plan to help us notice triggers and early warning signs as well as plan for things we can do each and every day to stay well and work toward our goals. (See Copeland, 2010 for more.) When developing your staying well plan, remember to keep handy a copy of your personal strengths, coping strategies, and resources list that you have been developing and adding to. You can put it in a purse or wallet or tape it to a wall or fridge where you can see it. Give a copy of your strengths, coping strategies, and resources list as well as your staying well plan to your family, friends, caregiver, clinician, and/or health care professional so they can help support your efforts and goals.

Noticing and Coping with Early Warning Signs

Early Warning Signs

Please list below your early warning signs:

1. _____

2. _____

3. _____

4. _____

5. _____

Please write down at least five things that are helpful for you to do when you notice early warning signs:

_____

_____

_____

_____

_____

Noticing and Coping with Triggers

Please write down your triggers:

_____

_____

_____

_____

Please write down coping strategies for triggers:

_____

_____

_____

_____

Things I Can Do to Stay Well

Please write down five to ten things that you can do to stay well:

_____

_____

_____

_____

Please write down ways you can give yourself a "pat on the back," to acknowledge all your efforts at staying well and working toward your goals. Remember it can be hard to do self-care on a regular basis; be kind and compassionate to yourself and celebrate your efforts!

_____

_____

_____

_____

_____

_____

Resources

We thank Julia Grummisch for her assistance in compiling this list. Please see http://www.treating psychosis.com for updates.

Psychosis Resources for Clinicians

Therapy for Psychosis

Beck, A. T., Rector, N. A., Stolar, N., & Grant, P. (2009). *Schizophrenia: Cognitive theory, research, and therapy.* New York, NY: Guilford Press.

Bellack, A. S., Mueser, K. T., Gingerich, S., & Agresta, J. (2004). *Social skills training for schizophrenia: A step-by-step guide.* New York, NY: Guilford Press.

Bentall, R. P. (2003). *Madness explained: Psychosis and human nature.* New York, NY: Penguin.

Byrne, S., Birchwood, M., Trower, P., & Meaden, A. (Eds.) (2006). *A casebook of cognitive behaviour therapy for command hallucinations: A social rank theory approach.* New York, NY: Routledge / Taylor & Francis Group.

Castle, D. J., Copolov, D. L., Wykes, T., & Mueser, K. T. (2012). *Pharmacological and psychosocial treatments in schizophrenia* (3rd ed.) Colchester, UK: Informa Healthcare.

Chadwick, P. (2006). *Person-based cognitive therapy for distressing psychosis.* Chichester, UK: John Wiley & Sons.

Chadwick, P., Birchwood, M., & Trower, P. (1996). *Cognitive therapy for delusions, voices, and paranoia.* Chichester, UK: John Wiley & Sons.

Chadwick, P. K. (2009). *Schizophrenia—The positive perspective: Explorations at the outer reaches of human experience.* New York, NY: Routledge / Taylor & Francis Group.

Clarke, I. (2010). *Psychosis and spirituality: Consolidating the new paradigm.* Chichester, UK: Wiley-Blackwell.

Cullberg, J. (2006). *Psychoses: An integrative perspective.* New York, NY: Routledge / Taylor & Francis Group.

Fowler, D., Garety, P., & Kuipers, L. (1995). *Cognitive therapy for psychosis.* Chichester, UK: Wiley.

Geekie, J., Randal, P., Lampshire, D., & Read, J. (2012). *Experiencing psychosis: Personal and professional perspectives.* New York, NY: Routledge / Taylor & Francis Group.

Gleeson, J. F. M., Killackey, E., & Krstev, H. (2008). *Psychotherapies for the psychoses: Theoretical, cultural, and clinical integration.* New York, NY: Routledge / Taylor & Francis Group.

Gumley, A., Gillham, A., Taylor, K, & Schwannauer, M. (2013). *Psychosis and emotion: The role of emotions in understanding psychosis, therapy, and recovery.* New York, NY: Routledge / Taylor & Francis Group.

Gumley, A., & Schwannauer, M. (2006). *Staying well after psychosis: A cognitive interpersonal approach to recovery and relapse prevention.* London, UK: John Wiley & Sons.

Hagen, R., Turkington, D., Berge, T., & Gråwe, R. W. (2011). *CBT for Psychosis: A symptom-based approach.* New York, NY: Routledge / Taylor & Francis Group.

Kingdon, D., & Turkington, D. (1994). *Cognitive-behavioral therapy of schizophrenia.* New York, NY: Guilford Press.

Kingdon, D., & Turkington, D. (Eds.). (2002). *The case study guide to cognitive behaviour therapy of psychosis.* Chichester, UK: John Wiley & Sons.

Kingdon, D. G., & Turkington, D. (2005). *Cognitive therapy of schizophrenia.* New York, NY: Guilford Press.

Laroi, F., & Aleman, A. (2010). *Hallucinations: A guide to treatment and management.* Oxford, UK: Oxford University Press.

McFarlane, W. R. (2002). *Multifamily groups in the treatment of severe psychiatric disorders.* New York, NY: Guilford Press.

Meaden, A., Keen, N., Aston, R., Barton, K., & Bucci, S. (2013). *Cognitive therapy for command hallucinations: An advanced practical companion.* London, UK: Routledge / Taylor & Francis Group.

Morris, E. M., Johns, L. C., & Oliver, J. E. (Eds.). (2013). *Acceptance and commitment therapy and mindfulness for psychosis.* Chichester, UK: Wiley-Blackwell.

Morrison, A. P. (Ed.). (2002). *A casebook of cognitive therapy for psychosis.* New York, NY: Brunner-Routledge.

Morrison, A. P., Renton, J. C., Dunn, H., Williams, S., & Bentall, R. P. (2004). *Cognitive therapy for psychosis: A formulation-based approach.* New York, NY: Brunner-Routledge.

Nelson, H. E. (2005). *Cognitive-behavioural therapy with delusions and hallucinations: A practice manual.* Cheltenham, UK: Nelson Thornes.

Perivoliotis, D., Grant, P., Beck, A. T., et al. (in press). *Recovery-oriented cognitive behavioral therapy for psychosis.* New York, NY: Guilford Press.

Read, J., & Dillon, J. (2013). *Models of madness: Psychological, social, and biological approaches to psychosis* (2nd ed.). London, UK: Routledge.

Rhodes, J., & Jakes, S. (2009). *Narrative CBT for psychosis.* New York, NY: Routledge / Taylor & Francis Group.

Sorensen, J. (2006). *Relapse prevention in schizophrenia and other psychoses: A treatment manual and workbook for therapist and client.* Hatfield, UK: University of Hertfordshire.

Steel, C. (Ed.). (2013). *CBT for schizophrenia: Evidence-based interventions and future directions.* Chichester, UK: John Wiley & Sons.

Tarrier, N., Gooding, P., Pratt, D., Kelly, J., Awenat, Y., & Maxwell, J. (2013). *Cognitive behavioural prevention of suicide in psychosis: A treatment manual.* London, UK: Routledge / Taylor & Francis Group.

Wright, J., Sudak, D. S., Turkington, D., & Thase, M. E. (2010). *High-yield cognitive-behavior therapy for brief sessions: An illustrated guide.* Arlington, VA: American Psychiatric Publishing

Wright, J. H., Turkington, D., Kingdon, D., & Basco, M. R. (2009). *Cognitive-behavior therapy for severe mental illness: An illustrated guide.* Arlington, VA: American Psychiatric Publishing.

Wykes, T., & Reeder, C. (2005). *Cognitive remediation therapy for schizophrenia: Theory and practice.* London, UK: Routledge / Taylor & Francis Group.

Early Psychosis/First Episode Psychosis

French, P., & Morrison, A. P. (2004). *Early detection and cognitive therapy for people at high risk of developing psychosis: A treatment approach.* Chichester, UK: John Wiley & Sons.

French, P., Smith, J., Shiers, D., Reed, M., & Rayne, M. (2010). *Promoting recovery in early psychosis: A practice manual.* Chichester, UK: John Wiley & Sons.

Gleeson, J. F. M., & McGorry P. D. (2004). *Psychological interventions in early psychosis: A treatment handbook.* Chichester, UK: John Wiley & Sons.

Jackson, H. J., & McGorry, P. D. (2009). *The recognition and management of early psychosis: A preventive approach* (2nd ed.). Cambridge, UK: Cambridge University Press.

Psychosis and Substance Use

Graham, H. L. (2004) *Cognitive-behavioural integrated treatment (C-BIT): A treatment manual for substance misuse in people with severe mental health problems.* Chichester, UK: John Wiley & Sons.

Graham, H. L., Copello, A., Birchwood, M. J., & Mueser, K. T. (2007) *Substance misuse in psychosis: Approaches to treatment and service delivery.* Chichester, UK: John Wiley & Sons.

Mueser, K. T., Noordsy, D. L., Drake, R. E., & Fox, L. (2003). *Integrated treatment for dual disorders: A guide to effective practice.* New York, NY: Guilford Press.

Psychosis and Trauma

Gold, S. N., & Elhai, J. D. (2008). *Trauma and serious mental illness.* Birmington, NY: Haworth Press.

Larkin, W., & Morrison, A. P. (Eds.). (2007). *Trauma and psychosis: New directions for theory and therapy.* New York, NY: Routledge.

Moskowitz, A., Schäfer, I., & Dorahy, M. J. (2009). *Psychosis, trauma, and dissociation: Emerging perspectives on severe psychopathology.* Chichester, UK: Wiley-Blackwell.

Recovery

Copeland, M. E. (2010). *WRAP Plus.* West Dummerston, VT: Peach Press.

Copeland, M., & Mead, S. (2004). *Wellness Recovery Action Plan & peer support: Personal, group, and program development.* West Dummerston, VT: Peach Press.

McNamara, S. (2009). *Voices of recovery.* Boston, MA: Center for Psychiatric Rehabilitation.

Ridgway, P., McDiarmid, D., Davidson, L., Bayes, J., & Ratzlaff, S. (2002). *Pathways to recovery: A strengths recovery self-help workbook.* Lawrence, KS: University of Kansas School of Social Welfare.

Psychosis Resources for Clients and Families

Freeman, D., Freeman, J., & Garety, P. (2008). *Overcoming paranoid and suspicious thoughts: A self-help guide using cognitive behavioral techniques.* New York, NY: Basic Books.

Hayward, M., Strauss, C., & Kingdon, D. (2012). *Overcoming distressing voices: A self-help guide using cognitive behavioral techniques.* London, UK: Constable & Robinson.

Lafond, V. (2002). *Grieving mental illness: A guide for patients and their caregivers.* Toronto, ON: University of Toronto Press.

Morrison, A. P., Renton, J. C., French, P., & Bentall, R. P. (2008). *Think you're crazy? Think again: A resource book for cognitive therapy for psychosis.* New York, NY: Routledge / Taylor & Francis Group.

Mueser, K. T., & Gingerich, S. (2006). *The complete family guide to schizophrenia.* New York, NY: Guilford Press.

Temes, R. (2002). *Getting your life back together when you have schizophrenia.* Oakland, CA: New Harbinger Publications.

Turkington, D., Kingdon, D., Rathod, S., Wilcock, S. K. J., Brabban, A., Cromarty, P., et al. (2009). *Back to life, back to normality.* Cambridge, UK: Cambridge University Press.

Resources for Clinicians, Clients, and Families

Application-Specific Resources

Brief Interventions

Altman, D. (2011). *One-minute mindfulness: 50 simple ways to find peace, clarity, and new possibilities in a stressed-out world.* Novato, CA: New World Library.

Davich, V. (2004). *8 minute meditation: Quiet your mind. Change your life.* New York, NY: Perigee.

Hawn, G., & Holden, W. (2011). *10 mindful minutes.* New York, NY: Perigee.

Kabat-Zinn, J. (2007). *Arriving at your own door: 108 lessons in mindfulness.* New York, NY: Hyperion.

Otto, M. W., Simon, N. M., Olatunji, B. O., Sung, S. C., & Pollack, M. H. (2011). *10-minute CBT: Integrating cognitive-behavioral strategies into your practice.* New York, NY: Oxford University Press.

Group Therapy

Bieling, P. J., McCabe, R. E., & Antony, M. M. (2006). *Cognitive-behavioral therapy in groups.* New York, NY: Guilford Press.

Yalom, I., D., & Leszcz, M. (2005). *The theory and practice of group psychotherapy* (5th ed.). New York, NY: Basic Books.

Orientation-Specific Resources

Acceptance and Commitment Therapy

Harris, R. (2007). *The happiness trap: How to stop struggling and start living.* Boston, MA: Trumpeter Books.

Harris, R. (2009). *ACT made simple.* Oakland, CA: New Harbinger Publications.

Harris, R. (2013). *Getting Unstuck in ACT: A clinician's guide to overcoming common obstacles in acceptance and commitment therapy.* Oakland, CA: New Harbinger Publications.

Hayes, S. C., Barnes-Holmes, D., & Roche, B. (2001). *Relational frame theory: A post-Skinnerian account of human language and cognition.* New York, NY: Plenum Press.

Hayes, S. C., Follette, V. M., & Linehan, M. M. (Eds.). (2011). *Mindfulness and acceptance: Expanding the cognitive-behavioral tradition.* New York, NY: Guilford Press.

Hayes, S. C., Strosahl, K. D., & Wilson, K. G. (2012). *Acceptance and commitment therapy: The process and practice of mindful change* (2nd ed.). New York, NY: Guilford.

Behavioral Activation

Addis, M. E., & Martell, C. R. (2004). *Overcoming depression one step at a time: The new behavioral activation approach to getting your life back.* Oakland, CA: New Harbinger Publications.

Kanter, J., Busch, A. M., & Rusch, L. C. (2009). *Behavioral activation: Distinctive features.* London, UK: Routledge.

Martell, C. R., Dimidjian, S., & Herman-Dunn, R. (2010). *Behavioral activation for depression: A clinician's guide.* New York, NY: Guilford Press.

Cognitive Behavioral Therapy

Bannink, F. (2010). *1001 solution-focused questions: Handbook for solution-focused interviewing.* New York, NY: W. W. Norton & Company.

Barlow, D. H., Farchione, T. J., Fairholme, C. P., Ellard, K. K., Boisseau, C. L., Allen, L. B., & Ehrenreich-May, J. (2011). *Unified protocol for transdiagnostic treatment of emotional disorders: Therapist guide.* New York, NY: Oxford University Press.

Beck, A. T. (1976). *Cognitive therapy and the emotional disorders.* New York, NY: International Universities Press.

Beck, J. S. (2005). *Cognitive therapy for challenging problems: What to do when the basics don't work.* New York, NY: Guilford Press.

Beck, J. S. (2011). *Cognitive behavior therapy: Basics and beyond* (2nd ed.). New York, NY: Guilford Press.

Bennett-Levy, J., Butler, G., Fennell, M., Hackmann, A., Mueller, M., & Westbrook, D. (2004). *Oxford guide to behavioural experiments in cognitive therapy.* Oxford, UK: Oxford University Press.

Fisher, P., & Wells, A. (2009). *Metacognitive therapy.* New York, NY: Routledge / Taylor & Francis Group.

Grawe, K. (2004). *Psychological therapy.* Cambridge, MA: Hogrefe & Huber Publishers.

Hackmann, A., Bennett-Levy, J., & Holmes, E. A. (2011). *Oxford guide to imagery in cognitive therapy.* Oxford, UK: Oxford University Press.

Leahy, R. L., Holland, S. J. F., & McGinn, L. K. (2012). *Treatment plans and interventions for depression and anxiety disorders* (2nd ed.). New York, NY: Guilford Press.

Mansell, W., Carey, T. A., & Tai, S. J. (2012). *A transdiagnostic approach to CBT using method of levels therapy: Distinctive features.* London, UK: Routledge / Taylor & Francis Group.

Newman, C. F. (2013). *Core competencies in cognitive-behavioural therapy: Becoming a highly effective and competent cognitive-behavioural therapist.* London, UK: Routledge.

Wells, A. (2000). *Emotional disorders and metacognition: Innovative cognitive therapy.* Chichester, UK: John Wiley & Sons.

Compassion-Focused Therapy and Self-Compassion

Germer, C. K. (2009). *The mindful path to self-compassion: Freeing yourself from destructive thoughts and emotions.* New York, NY: Guilford Press.

Gilbert, P. (2009). *The compassionate mind: A new approach to life's challenges.* London, UK: Constable & Robinson.

Gilbert, P. (2010). *Compassion-focused therapy.* New York, NY: Routledge / Taylor & Francis Group.

Gilbert, P., & Choden (2013). *Mindful compassion: Using the power of mindfulness and compassion to transform our lives.* London, UK: Constable & Robinson.

Kolts, R. L. (2012). *The compassionate-mind guide to managing your anger: Using compassion-focused therapy to calm your rage and heal your relationships.* Oakland, CA: New Harbinger Publications.

Neff, K. (2011). *Self-compassion: Stop beating yourself up and leave insecurity behind.* New York, NY: William Morrow.

Welford, M. (2012). *The compassionate mind approach to building your self-confidence using compassion-focused therapy.* London, UK: Constable & Robinson.

Welford, M. (2013). *The power of self-compassion: Using compassion-focused therapy to end self-criticism and build self-confidence.* Oakland, CA: New Harbinger Publications.

Emotion Regulation and Skills Training

Bein, A. (2013). *Dialectical behavior therapy for wellness and recovery: Interventions and activities for diverse client needs.* Hoboken, NJ: John Wiley & Sons.

Leahy, R. L., Tirch, D., & Napolitano, L. A. (2011). *Emotion regulation in psychotherapy: A practitioner's guide.* New York, NY: Guilford Press.

Linehan, M. M. (1993). *Skills training manual for treating borderline personality disorder.* New York, NY: Guilford Press.

McKay, M., Wood, J. C., & Brantley, J. (2007). *The dialectical behavior therapy skills workbook: Practical DBT exercises for learning mindfulness, interpersonal effectiveness, emotion regulation, and distress tolerance.* Oakland, CA: New Harbinger Publications.

Paterson, R. J. (2000). *The assertiveness workbook: How to express your ideas and stand up for yourself at work and in relationships.* Oakland, CA: New Harbinger Publications.

Mindfulness

Brach, T. (2004). *Radical acceptance: Embracing your life with the heart of a buddha.* New York, NY: Bantam.

Cayoun, B. (2011). *Mindfulness integrated CBT: Principles and practice.* Hoboken, NJ: Wiley-Blackwell.

Chodron, P. (2000). *When things fall apart: Heart advice for difficult times.* Boston, MA: Shambhala.

Germer, C. K., & Siegel, R. D. (2012). *Wisdom and compassion in psychotherapy: Deepening mindfulness in clinical practice.* New York, NY: Guilford Press.

Kabat-Zinn, J. (1990). *Full catastrophe living.* New York, NY: Dell Publishing.

Monteiro, L., & Musten, F. (2013). *Mindfulness starts here: An eight-week guide to skillful living.* Victoria, BC: FriesenPress.

Nhat Hanh, Thich. (1987). *The miracle of mindfulness: A manual on meditation.* (M. H., Trans.). Boston, MA: Beacon.

Salzberg, S. (1995). *Loving-kindness: The revolutionary art of happiness.* Boston, MA: Shambhala.

Siegel, R. D. (2010). *The mindfulness solution: Everyday practices for everyday problems.* New York, NY: Guilford Press.

Williams, J. M. G., & Kabat-Zinn, J. (2013). *Mindfulness: Diverse perspectives on its meaning, origins, and applications.* London, UK: Routledge.

Motivational Interviewing

Arkowitz, H., Westra, H. A., Miller, W. R., & Rollnick, S. (2007). *Motivational interviewing in the treatment of psychological problems.* New York, NY: Guilford Press.

Miller, W. R., & Rollnick, S. (2013). *Motivational interviewing: Helping people change* (3rd ed.). New York, NY: Guilford Press.

Positive Psychology

Fredrickson, B. L. (2009). *Positivity.* New York, NY: Three Rivers Press.

Hanson, R. (2009). *Buddha's brain: The practical neuroscience of happiness, love, and wisdom.* Oakland, CA: New Harbinger Publications.

Hanson, R. (2013). *Hardwiring happiness: The new brain science of contentment, calm, and confidence.* New York, NY: Harmony Books.

Lyubomirsky, S. (2007). *The how of happiness: A new approach to getting the life you want.* New York, NY: Penguin.

Seligman, M. E. P. (2004). *Authentic happiness: Using the new positive psychology to realize your potential for lasting fulfillment.* New York, NY: Atria Books.

Seligman, M. E. P. (2012). *Flourish: A visionary new understanding of happiness and well-being.* New York, NY: Atria Books.

Problem-Specific Resources

Anxiety Disorders (General)

Abramowitz, J. S., Deacon, B. J., & Whiteside, S. P. H. (2011). *Exposure therapy for anxiety: Principles and practice.* New York, NY: Guilford Press.

Antony, M. M., & Norton, P. J. (2008). *The anti-anxiety workbook: Proven strategies to overcome worry, phobias, panic, and obsessions.* New York, NY: Guilford Press.

Butler, G., Fennell, M., & Hackmann, A. (2008). *Cognitive-behavioral therapy for anxiety disorders: Mastering clinical challenges.* New York, NY: Guilford Press.

Clark, D. A., & Beck, A. T. (2010). *Cognitive therapy of anxiety disorders: Science and practice.* New York, NY: Guilford Press.

Clark, D. A., & Beck, A. T. (2012). *The anxiety and worry workbook: The cognitive behavioral solution.* New York, NY: Guilford Press.

Forsyth, J. P., & Eifert, G. H. (2008). *The mindfulness and acceptance workbook for anxiety: A guide to breaking free from anxiety, phobias, and worry using acceptance and commitment therapy.* Oakland, CA: New Harbinger Publications.

Tirch, D. D. (2012). *The compassionate-mind guide to overcoming anxiety: Using compassion-focused therapy to calm worry, panic, and fear.* Oakland, CA: New Harbinger Publications.

Depression

Greenberger, D., & Padesky, C. A. (1995). *Mind over mood: Change how you feel by changing the way you think.* New York, NY: Guilford Press.

Leahy, R. L. (2010). *Beat the blues before they beat you: How to overcome depression.* Carlsbad, CA: Hay House.

Otto, M., & Smits, J. (2011). *Exercise for mood and anxiety: Proven strategies for overcoming depression and enhancing well-being.* New York, NY: Oxford University Press.

Segal, Z. V., Williams, J. M. G., & Teasdale, J. D. (2002). *Mindfulness-based cognitive therapy for depression: A new approach to preventing relapse.* New York, NY: Guilford Press.

Zettle, R. D. (2007). *ACT for depression: A clinician's guide to using acceptance and commitment therapy in treating depression.* Oakland, CA: New Harbinger Publications.

Generalized Anxiety Disorder and Worry

Dugas, M. J., & Robichaud, M. (2006). *Cognitive-behavioral treatment for generalized anxiety disorder.* London, UK: Routledge.

Freeman, D., & Freeman, J. (2013). *How to keep calm and carry on: Inspiring ways to worry less and live a happier life*. Harlow, UK: Pearson.

Leahy, R. L. (2006). *The worry cure: Seven steps to stop worry from stopping you*. New York, NY: Crown Publishing.

Rygh, J. L., & Sanderson, W. C. (2004). *Treating generalized anxiety disorder: Evidence-based strategies, tools, and techniques*. New York, NY: Guilford Press.

Health Anxiety

Taylor, S., & Asmundson, G. J. G. (2004). *Treating health anxiety: A cognitive-behavioral approach*. New York, NY: Guilford Press.

Willson, R., & Veale, D. (2009). *Overcoming health anxiety: A self-help guide using cognitive behavioral techniques*. London, UK: Constable & Robinson.

Obsessive-Compulsive Disorder

Abramowitz, J. S. (2009). *Getting over OCD: A 10-step workbook for taking back your life*. New York, NY: Guilford Press.

Antony, M. M., Purdon, C., & Summerfeldt, L. J. (2006). *Psychological treatment of obsessive-compulsive disorder: Fundamentals and beyond*. Washington, DC: American Psychological Association.

Baer, L. (2002). *The imp of the mind: Exploring the silent epidemic of obsessive bad thoughts*. New York, NY: Penguin.

Panic Disorder and Agoraphobia

Barlow, D. H., & Craske, M. G. (2006). *Mastery of your anxiety and panic: Workbook* (4th ed.). Oxford, UK: Oxford University Press.

Craske, M. G., & Barlow, D. H. (2006). *Mastery of your anxiety and panic: Therapist guide* (4th ed.). Oxford, UK: Oxford University Press.

Sleep Problems

Davidson, J. R. (2012). *Sink into sleep: A step-by-step workbook for reversing insomnia*. New York, NY: Demos Medical Publishing.

Edinger, J. D., & Carney, C. E. (2008). *Overcoming insomnia: A cognitive-behavioral therapy approach—therapist guide*. Oxford, UK: Oxford University Press.

Edinger, J. D., & Carney, C. E. (2008). *Overcoming insomnia: A cognitive-behavioral therapy approach—workbook.* Oxford, UK: Oxford University Press.

Smoking Cessation

Hayes, S. C., & Levin, M. E. (2012). *Mindfulness and acceptance for addictive behaviors: Applying contextual CBT to substance abuse and behavioral addictions.* Oakland, CA: Context Press.

Perkins, K. A., Conklin, C. A., & Levine, M. D. (2007). *Cognitive-behavioral therapy for smoking cessation: A practical guidebook to the most effective treatments.* New York, NY: Routledge.

Social Anxiety

Antony, M. M., & Swinson, R. P. (2008). *The shyness and social anxiety workbook: Proven, step-by-step techniques for overcoming your fear* (2nd ed.). Oakland, CA: New Harbinger Publications.

Hofmann, S. G., & Otto, M. W. (2008). *Cognitive behavioral therapy for social anxiety disorder: Evidence-based and disorder-specific treatment techniques.* London, UK: Routledge.

Trauma-Related Problems

Briere, J., & Scott, C. (2012). *Principles of trauma therapy: A guide to symptoms, evaluation, and treatment* (2nd ed.). Thousand Oaks, CA: Sage Publications.

Cloitre, M., Cohen, L. R., & Koenen, K. C. (2006). *Treating survivors of childhood abuse: Psychotherapy for the interrupted life.* New York, NY: Guilford Press.

Courtois, C. A., & Ford, J. D. (2012). *Treatment of complex trauma: A sequenced, relationship-based approach.* New York, NY: Guilford Press.

Najavits, L. M. (2001). *Seeking safety: A treatment manual for PTSD and substance abuse.* New York, NY: Guilford Press.

Taylor, S. (2006). *Clinician's guide to PTSD: A cognitive-behavioral approach.* New York, NY: Guilford Press.

Walser, R. D., & Westrup, D. (2007). *Acceptance and commitment therapy for the treatment of post-traumatic stress disorder and trauma-related problems.* Oakland, CA: New Harbinger Publications.

Weight Management

Beck, J. S. (2007). *The Beck diet solution weight loss workbook.* Birmingham, AL: Oxmoor House.

Laliberte, M., McCabe, R. E., & Taylor, V. (2009). *The cognitive behavioral workbook for weight management: A step-by-step program.* Oakland, CA: New Harbinger Publications.

Other Useful Resources: Mobile Applications and Websites

Mobile Applications

CBT Referee

http://www.cbtreferee.com/

CBT Referee is a smartphone application that enables users to write down thoughts when they happen, in order to catch flawed thinking and learn from it. Users are able to invent their own referee who gives them a fair take on each thought.

LifeTick

http://www.lifetick.com/

LifeTick is a web-based application that facilitates goal setting. Its program follows the SMART goal-setting method—specific, measurable, achievable, realistic, time-limited—and creates tasks and reminders that give the user direction, purpose, and confidence in reaching new goals. It is also available on iPhone, iPad, and Android devices.

Live Happy

http://www.livehappyapp.com/

The Live Happy application was developed by Dr. Sonja Lyubomirsky and is described as a mobile happiness-boosting program. The application guides users through a set of daily activities intended to boost both short- and long-term happiness.

Mindfulness App

http://www.mindfulnessapp.com/

This mobile application integrates mindfulness-based approaches into its CBT program and is suitable for Apple and Android devices. It provides a variety of basic to advanced mindfulness approaches that vary in length and serves as a great tool for anyone.

Mindshift

http://www.anxietybc.com/mobile-app

This mobile application is designed to help teenagers and young adults cope with anxiety. It serves as a portable coach to help its users face challenging situations and take charge of their lives. It includes strategies to help deal with perfectionism, worry, panic, and conflict as well as test, social, and performance anxiety. It is available for download on Apple and Android devices.

MoodKit

http://www.thriveport.com/

This website is associated with the mobile application entitled MoodKit. With over two hundred mood improvement activities—complete with examples and tips, journal templates, customizable reminders, and recommended activities tailored to the user's individual needs—this program offers a step-by-step guidance experience to identify, evaluate, and modify thoughts to reduce distress.

Websites

Academy of Cognitive Therapy

http://www.academyofct.org

The Academy of Cognitive Therapy website provides resources on cognitive therapy, including cognitive therapy training and certification, a referral service for finding certified cognitive therapists, recommended reading and resources, as well as cognitive therapy rating scales and manuals.

Authentic Happiness

http://www.authentichappiness.sas.upenn.edu

This is the official website of Dr. Martin Seligman. He is the founder of positive psychology, which focuses on the empirical study of happiness and positive emotions. Among other resources, the website offers the VIA strengths questionnaire, a psychometric survey on character strengths and virtues.

Beck Institute of Cognitive Behavior Therapy

http://www.beckinstitute.org

This is the website of Dr. Aaron Beck (founder of CBT), Dr. Judith Beck, and the Beck Institute for Cognitive Behavior Therapy. It provides invaluable information and resources on international leadership, certified CBT therapists, and CBT training and education (including CBT workshops, tailored or specialized CBT training programs, and CBT supervision).

CBT Psychosis Online Training for Professionals

http://www.praxiscbtonline.co.uk

PraxisCBT is an online training program providing core training in CBT that is straightforward yet stimulating. Training may be completed as either (1) ongoing professional development or (2) for university credit up to postgraduate certificate.

Compassionate Mind Foundation

http://www.compassionatemind.co.uk

The Compassionate Mind Foundation was founded in 2006 by Dr. Paul Gilbert with the aim of promoting well-being through the scientific understanding and application of compassion. The website provides resources related to compassion-focused therapy including exercises, videos, and books.

Gloucestershire Hearing Voices and Recovery Groups

http://www.hearingvoices.org.uk/info_resources11.htm

The Gloucestershire Hearing Voices and Recovery Groups website is designed for individuals who hear voices and for people interested in helping others who hear voices. It provides information related to group work for people with psychosis as well as other information for clients and caregivers.

Good Days Ahead

http://www.mindstreet.com

Good Days Ahead is an online interactive program designed for individuals with depression and anxiety. It teaches individuals how to change negative thinking, control their moods, and use alternative methods to fight depression and anxiety. It incorporates videos, graphics, and self-help exercises to help make positive changes in how one thinks and feels.

Hanson, Dr. Rick

http://www.rickhanson.net

Dr. Rick Hanson is a neuropsychologist and author of *Buddha's Brain* and *Hardwiring Happiness*. This website provides resources on happiness, love, and wisdom.

Hearing Voices Network

http://www.hearing-voices.org

The Hearing Voices Network is meant for people who hear voices, see visions, or have other unusual perceptions. The organization promotes, develops, and supports self-help groups with the goal of raising awareness of voice hearing, visions, tactile sensations, and other sensory experiences. It allows everyone who has these experiences an opportunity to talk freely about them together in a compassionate environment.

Institute for Meditation and Psychotherapy

http://www.meditationandpsychotherapy.org

The Institute for Meditation and Psychotherapy offers training for professionals, including exploration of the integration of mindfulness and psychotherapy as well as personal enrichment by deepening your practice in your life and livelihood. It also encourages shared community by connecting clinicians with like-minded colleagues and practitioners.

Mental Wellness Today

http://www.mentalwellnesstoday.com

This website provides resources on mental health—including information on *SZ Magazine,* which was founded by Bill McPhee and provides information and resources related to schizophrenia-spectrum disorders and psychosis for consumers, clients, and families.

Mind

http://www.mind.org.uk

Mind is a mental health charity aimed at providing support for those experiencing a mental health problem. The website has a vast store of information for those living with a mental health problem and for those supporting someone who is. The website also allows for its users to get involved and learn about Mind's new events and campaigns, and it links them to its helpline.

Mindful Self-Compassion

http://www.MindfulSelfCompassion.org

Mindful Self-Compassion is operated by Dr. Christopher Germer, a clinical psychologist specializing in mindfulness and compassion-based psychotherapy. His website includes news on recent workshops, instructions for meditation and psychotherapy, handouts, and more.

MoodGYM Training Program

http://www.moodgym.anu.edu.au

The MoodGYM is a training program designed to help individuals learn cognitive behavior therapy skills for preventing and coping with depression. With over 600,000 registered users, this popular Australian-based online program consists of five modules, an interactive game, anxiety and depression assessments, downloadable relaxation audio, a workbook, and feedback assessment.

National Alliance on Mental Illness (information and support)

http://www.nami.org

The National Alliance on Mental Illness (NAMI) website provides a wide variety of help, including information regarding mental illnesses, treatments, finding the closest NAMI organization/affiliates to you, and more.

Neff, Dr. Kristin

See Self-Compassion (below).

Outcome Measures

http://www.outcometracker.org

This website provides a list of outcome measures that are available free of charge.

Paranoid Thoughts

http://www.paranoidthoughts.com

This website is about unfounded or excessive fears about others—specifically, paranoid thoughts and paranoia. Based on the book by Daniel Freeman and colleagues, *Overcoming Paranoid and Suspicious Thoughts*, the website provides information about coping with paranoia, getting help, and becoming happy.

Rethink

http://www.rethink.org/

Rethink is a very useful website based out of the UK with numerous resources for individuals experiencing schizophrenia. It promotes the rethinking of mental illness and provides useful information for caregivers, family, friends, and individuals living with schizophrenia.

SANE (information and support)

http://www.sane.org.uk

The SANE website provides direct help with social support, offers information about the challenges of mental illnesses, and raises awareness.

Self-Compassion

http://www.self-compassion.org

This website, by Dr. Kristin Neff, provides information about self-compassion intended for students, researchers, and the general public. Video and audio clips related to self-compassion, self-kindness, common humanity, mindfulness, and self-compassion vs. self-esteem are available free of charge, as are other useful resources and exercises.

Sleep Improvement

http://www.cbtforinsomnia.com

This website is dedicated to treating insomnia through the use of CBT. It has both an online program and a CD-based program that have been shown to improve insomnia. Other information related to sleep disturbances is available at http://www.helpguide.org/life/insomnia_treatment.htm

Sounds True

http://www.soundstrue.com

This website is dedicated to sharing spiritual resources via video and audio recordings of a wide variety of spiritual teachings, music, guided meditations, exercises, interviews with spiritual teachers, and so on. The site also hosts a blog and publishes a weekly e-newsletter, which includes free teachings.

This Way Up Clinic

https://www.thiswayup.org.au/clinic/

This Way Up Clinic is a clinician-guided, evidence-based program out of Australia that offers courses and support for a fee. Clients work with clinicians who will monitor their progress and offer effective treatments for combating their anxiety or depression.

Treating Psychosis

http://www.treatingpsychosis.com

This is the website associated with this book, *Treating Psychosis*. The website features resources including useful websites, books, videos, handouts, as well as other supplemental information relating to psychosis, including additional chapters on treating anxiety and trauma.

Virtual Reality Programs

http://www.virtuallybetter.com

Virtually Better is a clinic that specializes in the use of CBT and brings interactive technology to behavioral health care for treatment and training. The clinic provides services to children, adolescents, and families faced with emotional and behavioral difficulties as well as to adults who struggle to cope with everyday emotional, occupational, and relationship issues. It also uses evidence-based virtual reality exposure for phobias, addiction, skills development, PTSD, and stress management.

Reference List

Abba, N., Chadwick, P. D. J., & Stevenson, C. (2008). Responding mindfully to distressing psychosis: A grounded theory analysis. *Psychotherapy Research, 18,* 77–87. doi:10.1080/10503300701367992

Ali, S., Patel, M., Avenido, J., Bailey, R. K., Jabeen, S., & Riley, W. J. (2011). Hallucinations: Common features and causes. *Current Psychiatry, 10,* 22–26.

Alloway, T. P. (2011). A comparison of working memory profiles in children with ADHD and DCD. *Child Neuropsychology, 17,* 483–494.

American Psychiatric Association. (2013). *Diagnostic and statistical manual of mental disorders* (5th ed.), Washington, DC: Author.

Bach, P., & Hayes, S. C. (2002). The use of acceptance and commitment therapy to prevent the rehospitalization of psychotic patients: A randomized controlled trial. *Journal of Consulting and Clinical Psychology, 70,* 1129–1139. doi:10.1037//0022006X.70.5.1129

Bach, P., Hayes, S. C., & Gallop, R. (2012). Long-term effects of brief acceptance and commitment therapy for psychosis. *Behavior Modification, 36,* 165–181. doi:10.1177/0145445511427193

Barlow, D. H. (2002). *Anxiety and its disorders: The nature and treatment of anxiety and panic* (2nd ed.). New York, NY: Guilford Press.

Barlow, D. H., Farchione, T. J., Fairholme, C. P., Ellard, K. K., Boisseau, C. L., Allen, L. B., & Ehrenreich-May, J. (2011). *The unified protocol for transdiagnostic treatment of emotional disorders: Therapist guide.* New York, NY: Oxford University Press.

Beck, A. T. (1970). *Depression: Causes and treatment.* Philadelphia, PA: University of Pennsylvania Press.

Beck, A. T., Rector, N. A., Stolar, N., & Grant, P. (2009). *Schizophrenia: Cognitive theory, research, and therapy.* New York, NY: Guilford Press.

Beck, A. T., Rush, A. J., Shaw, B. F., & Emery, G. (1979). *Cognitive therapy of depression.* New York, NY: Guilford Press.

Beck, J. S. (1995). *Cognitive therapy: Basics and beyond.* New York, NY: Guilford Press.

Beck, J. S. (2011). *Cognitive behavior therapy: Basics and beyond* (2nd ed.). New York, NY: Guilford Press.

Bendall, S., McGorry, P., & Krstev, H. (2006). The trauma of being psychotic. In W. Larkin & A. P. Morrison (Eds.), *Trauma and psychosis: New directions for theory and therapy* (pp. 58–74). New York, NY: Routledge.

Bentall, R. P. (2004). *Madness explained: Psychosis and human nature.* London, UK: Penguin.

Bentall, R. P., Rowse, G., Shrayne, N., Kinderman, P., Howard, R., Blackwood, N., et al. (2009). The cognitive and affective structure of paranoid delusions: A transdiagnostic investigation of patients with schizophrenia spectrum disorders and depression. *Archives of General Psychiatry, 66,* 236–247. doi:10.1001/archgenpsychiatry.2009.1

Bernstein, E. M., & Putnam, F. W. (1986). Development, reliability, and validity of a dissociation scale. *The Journal of Nervous and Mental Disease, 174,* 727–735.

Birchwood, M., Meaden, A., Trower, P., Gilbert, P., & Plaistow, J. (2000). The power and omnipotence of voices: Subordination and entrapment by voices and significant others. *Psychological medicine, 30,* 337–344.

Braehler, C., Gumley, A., Harper, J., Wallace, S., Norrie, J., & Gilbert, P. (2013). Exploring change processes in compassion focused therapy in psychosis: Results of a feasibility randomized controlled trial. *British Journal of Clinical Psychology, 52,* 199–214. doi:10.1111/bjc.12009

Braehler, C., Harper, J., & Gilbert, P. (2013). Compassion focused group therapy for recovery after psychosis. In C. Steel (Ed.), *CBT for schizophrenia: Evidence-based interventions and future directions.* Chichester, U.K.: Wiley-Blackwell.

Byrne, S., Birchwood, M., Trower, P. E., & Meaden, A. (2006). *A casebook of cognitive behaviour therapy for command hallucinations: A social rank theory approach.* Hove, UK: Psychology Press.

Canadian Psychiatric Association. (2005). Clinical practice guidelines: Treatment of schizophrenia. *Canadian Journal of Psychiatry, 50*(S1), 7s–57s.

Chadwick, P. K. (2006). How social difficulties produce cognitive problems during the mediation of psychosis: A qualitative study. *International Journal of Social Psychiatry, 52,* 459–468.

Chadwick, P., Hughes, S., Russell, D., Russell, I., & Dagnan, D. (2009). Mindfulness groups for distressing voices and paranoia: A replication and randomized feasibility trial. *Behavioural and Cognitive Psychotherapy, 37,* 403–412. doi:10.1017/S1352465809990166

Chadwick, P., Lees, S., & Birchwood, M. (2000). The revised Beliefs About Voices Questionnaire (BAVQ-R). *The British Journal of Psychiatry, 177,* 229–232.

Chadwick, P., Newman-Taylor, K., & Abba, N. (2005). Mindfulness groups for people with psychosis. *Behavioural and Cognitive Psychotherapy, 33,* 351–359. doi:10.1017/S1352465805002158

Ciarrochi, J., Robb, H., & Godsell, C. (2005). Letting a little nonverbal air into the room: Insights from acceptance and commitment therapy. Part 1: Philosophical and theoretical underpinnings. *Journal of Rational-Emotive & Cognitive-Behavior Therapy, 23,* 79–106. doi:10.1007/s10942-005-0005-y

Coleman, R., & Smith, M. (2007). *Working with voices: Victim to victor* (2nd ed.) Peoria, IL: P&P Press.

Copeland, M. E. (2010). *WRAP Plus.* West Dummerston, VT: Peach Press.

Courtois, C. A., & Ford, J. D. (2012). *Treatment of complex trauma: A sequenced, relationship-based approach.* New York, NY: Guilford Press.

Eifert, G. H., & Forsyth, J. P. (2005). *Acceptance and commitment therapy for anxiety disorders: A practitioner's treatment guide to using mindfulness, acceptance, and values-based behavior change strategies.* Oakland, CA: New Harbinger Publications.

Fish, T. J. (1962). *Schizophrenia.* Baltimore, MD: Williams and Wilkins.

Folkman. S., & Lazarus, R. S. (1988). *Manual for the Ways of Coping Questionnaire*. Palo Alto, CA: Consulting Psychologists Press.

Fredrickson, B. L. (1998). What good are positive emotions? *Review of General Psychology, 2*, 300–319. doi:10.1037/1089-2680.2.3.300

Fredrickson, B. L. (2001). The role of positive emotions in positive psychology. *American Psychologist, 56*, 218–226. doi:10.1037/0003-066X.56.3.218

Freeman, D. (2011). Improving cognitive treatments for delusions. *Schizophrenia Research, 132*, 135–139.

Freeman, D., Brugha, T., Meltzer, H., Jenkins, R., Stahl, D., & Bebbington, P. (2010). Persecutory ideation and insomnia: Findings from the second British National Survey of Psychiatric Morbidity. *Journal of Psychiatric Research, 44*, 1021–1026.

French, P., & Morrison, A. P. (2004). *Early detection and cognitive therapy for people at high risk of developing psychosis: A treatment approach*. Chichester, UK: John Wiley & Sons.

Freud, S. (1959). Formulations regarding the two principles in mental functioning. In J. Strachey (Ed.), *Collected Papers*: Vol. 4 (pp. 13–21).

Garety, P. A., Kuipers, E., Fowler, D., Freeman, D., & Bebbington, P. E. (2001). A cognitive model of the positive symptoms of psychosis. *Psychological Medicine, 31*, 189–195. doi:10.1017/ S0033291701003312

Garis, R. I., & Farmer, K. C. (2002). Examining costs of chronic conditions in a Medicaid population. *Managed Care, 11*(3), 43–50.

Gaudiano, B. A., & Herbert, J. D. (2006). Believability of hallucinations as a potential mediator of their frequency and associated distress in psychotic inpatients. *Behavioural and Cognitive Psychotherapy, 34*, 497–502. doi:10.1017/S1352465806003080

Gaudiano, B. A., Herbert, J. D., & Hayes, S. C. (2010) Is it the symptom or the relation to it? Investigating potential mediators of change in acceptance and commitment therapy for psychosis. *Behavior Therapy, 41*, 543–554. doi:10.1016/j.beth.2010.03.001

Germer, C. K. (2009). *The mindful path to self-compassion: Freeing yourself from destructive thoughts and emotions*. New York, NY: Guilford Press.

Gilbert, P. (1992). *Depression: The evolution of powerlessness*. Hove, UK: Lawrence Erlbaum.

Gilbert, P. (2009). *The compassionate mind: A new approach to life's challenges*. Oakland, CA: New Harbinger Publications.

Gilbert, P. (2010). *Compassion-focused therapy*. New York, NY: Routledge / Taylor and Francis Group.

Gilbert, P., & Choden (2013). Mindful Compassion: Using the power of mindfulness and compassion to transform our lives. London, UK: Constable & Robinson.

Gilbert, P., Birchwood, M., Gilbert, J., Trower, P., Hay, J., Murray, B., Meaden, A., & Olsen, K. (2001). An exploration of evolved mental mechanisms for dominant and subordinate behaviour in relation to auditory hallucinations in schizophrenia and critical thoughts in depression. *Psychological Medicine, 31*, 1117–1127. doi:10.1017/S0033291701004093

Gortner, E. T., Gollan, J. K., Dobson, K. S., & Jacobson, N. S. (1998). Cognitive-behavioral treatment for depression: Relapse prevention. *Journal of Consulting and Clinical Psychology, 66*, 377–384. doi:10.1037/ 0022-006X.66.2.377

Grant, P. M., Huh, G. A., Perivoliotis, D., Stolar, N. M., & Beck, A. T. (2012). Randomized trial to evaluate the efficacy of cognitive therapy for low-functioning patients with schizophrenia. *Archives of General Psychiatry, 69*, 121–127.

Greenberg, J. S., Greenley, J. R., McKee, D., Brown, R., & Griffin-Francell, C. (1993). Mothers caring for an adult child with schizophrenia: The effects of subjective burden on maternal health. *Family Relations*, 205–211.

Greenberger, D., & Padesky, C. A. (1995). *Mind over mood: Change how you feel by changing the way you think.* New York, NY: Guilford Press.

Gumley, A., Birchwood, M., Fowler, D., & Gleeson, J. (2006). Individual psychological approaches to recovery and staying well after psychosis. *Acta Psychiatrica Scandinavica, 114,* 27.

Gumley, A., Braehler, C., Laithwaite, H., MacBeth, A., & Gilbert, P. (2010). A compassion focused model of recovery after psychosis. *International Journal of Cognitive Therapy, 3,* 186-201. doi:10.3410/f.14208966.15726073

Gumley, A., Gillham, A., Taylor, K., & Schwannauer, M. (2013). *Psychosis and emotion: The role of emotions in understanding psychosis, therapy, and recovery.* New York, NY: Routledge / Taylor & Francis Group.

Gumley, A., & Schwannauer, M. (2006). *Staying well after psychosis: A cognitive interpersonal approach to recovery and relapse prevention.* London, UK: John Wiley & Sons.

Haddock, G., McCarron, J., Tarrier, N., & Faragher, E. B. (1999). Scales to measure dimensions of hallucinations and delusions: The Psychotic Symptom Rating Scales (PSYRATS). *Psychological Medicine, 29,* 879–889.

Hanson, R. (2009). *Buddha's brain: The practical neuroscience of happiness, love, and wisdom.* Oakland, CA: New Harbinger Publications.

Hanson, R. (2013). *Hardwiring happiness: The new brain science of contentment, calm, and confidence.* New York, NY: Harmony.

Harris, R. (2007). *The happiness trap: How to stop struggling and start living.* Boston, MA: Trumpeter Books.

Harris, R. (2009). *ACT made simple.* Oakland, CA: New Harbinger Publications.

Hayes, S. C. (2004). Acceptance and commitment therapy and the new behavior therapies: Mindfulness, acceptance, and relationship. In S. C. Hayes, V. M. Follette, & M. Linehan (Eds.), *Mindfulness and acceptance: Expanding the cognitive-behavioral tradition* (pp. 1–29). New York, NY: Guilford Press.

Hayes, S. C., Luoma, J., Bond, F., Masuda, A., & Lillis, J. (2006). Acceptance and commitment therapy: Model, processes, and outcomes. *Behaviour Research and Therapy, 44,* 1–25. doi:10.1016/j.brat.2005.06.006

Hayes, S. C., Strosahl, K., & Wilson, K. G. (1999). *Acceptance and commitment therapy: An experiential approach to behavior change.* New York, NY: Guilford Press.

Hayes, S. C., Strosahl, K., & Wilson, K. G. (2012). *Acceptance and commitment therapy: The process and practice of mindful change* (2nd ed.). New York, NY: Guilford Press.

Hayes, S. C., Wilson, K. W., Gifford, E. V., Follette, V. M., & Strosahl, K. (1996). Experiential avoidance and behavioral disorders: A functional dimensional approach to diagnosis and treatment. *Journal of Consulting and Clinical Psychology, 64,* 1152–1168. doi:10.1037//0022-006X.64.6.1152

Hofmann, S. G., & Asmundson, G. J. (2008). Acceptance and mindfulness-based therapy: New wave or old hat? *Clinical Psychology Review, 28,* 1–16. doi:10.1016/j.cpr.2007.09.003

Hogg, L. (1996) Psychological treatments for negative symptoms. In G. Haddock & P. D. Slade (Eds.), *Cognitive-behavioural interventions in psychotic disorders* (pp. 151–167). London, UK: Routledge.

Hölzel, B. K., Lazar, S. W., Gard, T., Schuman-Olivier, Z., Vago, D. R., & Ott, U. (2011). How does mindfulness meditation work? Proposing mechanisms of action from a conceptual and neural perspective. *Perspectives on Psychological Science, 6,* 537–559.

Hopko, D. R., Lejuez, C. W., Ruggiero, K. J., & Eifert, G. H. (2003). Contemporary behavioral activation treatments for depression: Procedures, principles, and progress. *Clinical Psychology Review, 23,* 699–717.

Howard, A., Forsyth, A., Spencer, H., Young, E. W., & Turkington, D. (2013). Do voice hearers naturally use focusing and metacognitive coping techniques? *Psychosis, 5,* 119–126.

Jacobson, N. S., Dobson, K. S., Truax, P. A., Addis, M. E., Koerner, K., Gollan, J. K., et al. (1996). A component analysis of cognitive-behavioral treatment for depression. *Journal of Consulting and Clinical Psychology, 64,* 295–304. doi:10.1037/0022-006X.70.2.288

Kabat-Zinn, J. (1990). *Full catastrophe living: Using the wisdom of your mind to face stress, pain, and illness.* New York, NY: Dell Publishing.

Kabat-Zinn, J. (2003). Mindfulness-based interventions in context: Past, present, and future. *Clinical Psychology: Science and Practice, 10,* 144–156.

Kanter, J. W., Busch, A. M., & Rusch, L. C. (2009). *Behavioral activation: Distinctive features.* London, UK: Routledge.

Kent, M., & Davis, M. (2010). The emergence of capacity-building programs and models of resilience. In J. W. Reich, A. J. Zautra, & J. S. Hall (Eds.), *Handbook of adult resilience* (pp. 427–449). New York, NY: Guilford Press.

Khoury, B., & Lecomte, T. (2012). Emotion regulation and schizophrenia. *International Journal of Cognitive Therapy, 5,* 67–76. doi:10.1521/ijct.2012.5.1.67

Kingdon, D. G., & Turkington, D. (1991). Preliminary report: The use of cognitive behavior therapy and a normalizing rationale in schizophrenia. *Journal of Nervous and Mental Disease, 179,* 207–211.

Kingdon, D. G., & Turkington, D. (1994). *Cognitive-behavioral therapy of schizophrenia.* New York, NY: Guilford Press.

Kingdon, D. G., & Turkington, D. (2005). *Cognitive therapy of schizophrenia: Guides to individual treatment.* New York, NY: Guilford Press.

Kirkbride, J. B., & Jones, P. B. (2011). The prevention of schizophrenia—What can we learn from eco-epidemiology? *Schizophrenia Bulletin, 37*(2): 262-271.

Laithwaite, H., O'Hanlon, M., Collins, P., Doyle, P., Abraham, L., Porter, S., et al. (2009). Recovery After Psychosis (RAP): A compassion focused programme for individuals residing in high security settings. *Behavioural and Cognitive Psychotherapy, 37,* 511–526. doi:10.1017/S1352465809990233

Langer, A. I., Cangas, A. J., Salcedo, E., & Fuentes, B. (2012). Applying mindfulness therapy in a group of psychotic individuals: A controlled study. *Behavioural and Cognitive Psychotherapy, 40,* 105–109. doi:10.1017/S1352465811000464

Langer, A. I., Cangas, A. J., & Serper, M. (2011). Analysis of the multidimensionality of hallucination-like experiences in clinical and nonclinical Spanish samples and their relation to clinical symptoms: Implications for the model of continuity. *International Journal of Psychology, 46,* 46–54.

Laursen, T. M. (2011). Life expectancy among persons with schizophrenia or bipolar affective disorder. *Schizophrenia Research, 131,* 101–104. doi:10.1016/j.schres.2011.06.008

Leahy, R. L. (2003). *Cognitive therapy techniques: A practitioner's guide.* New York, NY: Guilford Press.

Leahy, R. L., Tirch, D., & Napolitano, L. A. (2011). *Emotion regulation in psychotherapy: A practitioner's guide.* New York, NY: Guilford Press.

Lejuez, C. W., Hopko, D. R., Acierno, R., Daughters, S. B., & Pagoto, S. L. (2011). Ten year revision of the brief behavioral activation treatment for depression: Revised treatment manual [Supplemental online materials]. *Behavior Modification, 35,* 111–161. doi: 10.1177/0145445510390929

Lejuez, C. W., Hopko, D. R., & Hopko, S. D. (2001). A brief behavioral activation treatment for depression: Treatment manual. *Behavior Modification, 25,* 255–286.

Linehan, M. M. (1993). *Cognitive-behavioral treatment of borderline personality disorder.* New York, NY: Guilford Press.

Linscott, R. J., & van Os, J. (2010). Systematic reviews of categorical versus continuum models in psychosis: Evidence for discontinuous subpopulations underlying a psychometric continuum—Implications for DSM–V, DSM–VI, and DSM–VII. *Annual Review of Clinical Psychology, 6,* 391–419. doi:10.1146/annurev.clinpsy.032408.153506

Mairs, H., Lovell, K., Campbell, M., & Keeley, P. (2011). Development and pilot investigation of behavioral activation for negative symptoms. *Behavior Modification, 35,* 486–506. doi:10.1177/0145445511411706

McFarlane, W. R. (2002). *Multifamily groups in the treatment of severe psychiatric disorders.* New York, NY: Guilford Press.

Meaden, A., Keen, N., Aston, R., Barton, K., & Bucci, S. (2013). *Cognitive therapy for command hallucinations: An advanced practical companion.* London, UK: Routledge / Taylor & Francis Group.

Moorhead, S., & Turkington, D. (2001). The CBT of delusional disorder: The relationship between schema vulnerability and psychotic content. *British Journal of Medical Psychology, 74,* 419–430. doi:10.1348/000711201161073

Morrison, A. P. (2001). The interpretation of intrusions in psychosis: An integrative cognitive approach to hallucinations and delusions. *Behavioural and Cognitive Psychotherapy, 29,* 257–276. doi:10.1017/S1352465801003010

Morrison, A. P., Renton, J. C., French, P., & Bentall, R. P. (2008). *Think you're crazy? Think again: A resource book for cognitive therapy for psychosis.* New York, NY: Routledge / Taylor & Francis Group.

Morrison, A. P., Turkington, D., Wardle, M., Spencer, H., Barratt, S., Dudley, R., et al. (2012). A preliminary exploration of predictors of outcome and cognitive mechanisms of change in cognitive behaviour therapy for psychosis in people not taking antipsychotic medication. *Behaviour Research and Therapy, 50,* 163–167.

Myers, E., Startup, H., & Freeman, D. (2013) Improving sleep, improving delusions: CBT for insomnia in individuals with persecutory delusions. In Craig Steel (Ed.), *CBT for schizophrenia: Evidence-based interventions and future directions* (pp. 213–233). Hoboken, NJ: John Wiley & Sons.

National Institute for Health and Care Excellence (NICE). (2009). *Core interventions in the treatment and management of schizophrenia in primary and secondary care.* Retrieved from http://www.nice.org.uk.

Neff, K. (2011). *Self-compassion: Stop beating yourself up and leave insecurity behind.* New York, NY: William Morrow.

Nhat Hanh, Thich. (1987). *The miracle of mindfulness.* Trans. M. Ho. Boston, MA: Beacon.

Opler, L. A., Kay, S. R., Lindenmayer, J., & Fiszbein, A. (1992). *SCI-PANSS.* Toronto, ON: Multi-Health Systems, Inc.

Otto, M., & Smits, J. (2011). *Exercise for mood and anxiety: Proven strategies for overcoming depression and enhancing well-being.* New York, NY: Oxford University Press.

Peterson, C., & Seligman, M. E. (2004). *Character strengths and virtues: A handbook and classification.* New York, NY: Oxford University Press.

Rabinowitz, J., De Smedt, G., Harvey, P. D., & Davidson, M. (2002). Relationship between premorbid functioning and symptom severity as assessed at first episode of psychosis. *American Journal of Psychiatry, 159,* 2021–2026.

Rath, T. (2007). *Strengths Finder 2.0.* New York, NY: Gallup Press.

Rathod, S., Kingdon, D., Smith, P., & Turkington, D. (2005) Insight into schizophrenia: The effects of cognitive behavioural therapy on the components of insight and association with sociodemographics—Data on a previously published randomised controlled trial. *Schizophrenia Research, 74,* 211–219.

Rector, N., & Beck, A. (2002). Cognitive therapy for schizophrenia: From conceptualization to intervention. *The Canadian Journal of Psychiatry, 47,* 41–50.

Robinson, D. G., Woerner, M. G., McMeniman, M., Mendelowitz, A., & Bilder, R. M. (2004). Symptomatic and functional recovery from a first episode of schizophrenia or schizoaffective disorder. *American Journal of Psychiatry, 161*, 473–479. doi:10.1176/appi.ajp.161.3.473

Schäfer, I., & Fisher, H. L. (2011). Childhood trauma and posttraumatic stress disorder in patients with psychosis: Clinical challenges and emerging treatments. *Current Opinion in Psychiatry, 24*, 514–518. doi:10.1097/YCO.0b013e32834b56c8

Segal, Z. V., Williams, J. M. G., & Teasdale, J. D. (2002). *Mindfulness-based cognitive therapy for depression: A new approach to preventing relapse.* New York, NY: Guilford Press.

Segal, Z. V., Williams, J. M. G., & Teasdale, J. D. (2012). *Mindfulness-based cognitive therapy for depression* (2nd ed.). New York, NY: Guilford Press.

Seligman, M. E. (2002). *Authentic happiness: Using the new positive psychology to realize your potential for lasting fulfillment.* New York, NY: The Free Press, Simon & Schuster.

Siegel, R. D. (2010). *The mindfulness solution: Everyday practices for everyday problems.* New York, NY: Guilford Press.

Sims, A. (1988). *Symptoms in the mind.* London, UK: Balliere Tindall.

Snyder, C. R., & Lopez, S. J. (Eds.). (2002). *Handbook of positive psychology.* New York, NY: Oxford University Press.

Tai, S., & Turkington, D. (2009). The evolution of cognitive behavior therapy for schizophrenia: Current practice and recent developments. *Schizophrenia Bulletin, 35*, 865–873. doi:10.1093/schbul/sbp080

Tarrier, N., Gooding, P., Pratt, D., Kelly, J., Awenat, Y., & Maxwell, J. (2013). *Cognitive behavioural prevention of suicide in psychosis: A treatment manual.* London, UK: Routledge / Taylor & Francis Group.

Teasdale, J. D., Segal, Z. V., & Williams, J. M. G. (1995). How does cognitive therapy prevent depressive relapse and why should attentional control (mindfulness) training help? *Behaviour Research and Therapy, 33*, 25–39. doi:10.1016/0005-7

Teasdale, J. D., Segal, Z. V., Williams, J. M. G., Ridgeway, V. A., Soulsby, J. M., & Lau, M. A. (2000). Prevention of relapse/recurrence in major depression by mindfulness-based cognitive therapy. *Journal of Consulting and Clinical Psychology, 68*, 615–623. doi:10.1037//0022-006X.68.4.615

Tirch, D. D. (2012). *The compassionate-mind guide to overcoming anxiety: Using compassion-focused therapy to calm worry, panic, and fear.* Oakland, CA: New Harbinger Publications.

Tirch, D., Schoendorff, B., & Silberstein, S. (in press). *The ACT Practitioner's Guide to the Science of Compassion.* Oakland, CA: New Harbinger Publications.

Trower, P., Birchwood, M., Meaden, A., Byrne, S., Nelson, A., & Ross, K. (2004). Cognitive therapy for command hallucinations: Randomised controlled trial. *The British Journal of Psychiatry, 184*, 312–320.

Turkington, D., Kingdon, D., Rathod, S., Wilcock, S. K. J., Brabban, A., Cromarty, P., et al. (2009). *Back to life, back to normality.* Cambridge, UK: Cambridge University Press.

Turkington, D., John, C. H., Siddle, R., Ward, D., & Birmingham, L. (1996). Cognitive therapy in the treatment of drug-resistant delusional disorder. *Clinical Psychology and Psychotherapy, 3*, 118–128. doi:10.1002/(SICI)1099-0879(199606)3:2<118::AID-CPP75>3.0.CO;2-R

Van der Gaag, M., Nieman, D., & van den Berg, D. (2013). *CBT for those at risk of a first-episode psychosis: Evidence-based psychotherapy for those with an "at risk mental state."* Hove, UK: Routledge.

van Os, J., & Linscott, R. J. (2012). Introduction: The extended psychosis phenotype—Relationship with schizophrenia and with ultrahigh risk status for psychosis. *Schizophrenia Bulletin, 38*, 227–230.

Welford, M. (2012). *The compassionate mind approach to building your self-confidence using compassion focused therapy.* London, UK: Constable & Robinson.

Weiden, P. J., & Turkington, D. (2012). Assessment and management of medication nonadherence in schizophrenia. In J. A. Lieberman & R. M. Murray (Eds.), *Comprehensive care of schizophrenia: A textbook of clinical management* (2nd ed., pp. 219–243). New York, NY: Oxford University Press.

Wells, A. (1994). Attention and the control of worry. In G. C. L. Davey & F. Tallis (Eds.), *Worrying: Perspectives on theory, assessment, and treatment* (pp. 91–114). Oxford, UK: Wiley.

Wells, A. (2000). *Emotional disorders and metacognition: Innovative cognitive therapy.* Chichester, UK: John Wiley & Sons.

Wells, A., & Matthews, G. (1994). *Attention and emotion: A clinical perspective.* Hove, UK: Lawrence Erlbaum.

White, R. G., Gumley, A. I., McTaggart, J., Rattrie, L., McConville, D., Cleare, S., & Mitchell, G. (2011). A feasibility study of acceptance and commitment therapy for emotional dysfunction following psychosis. *Behaviour Research and Therapy, 49,* 901–907. doi:10.1016/j.brat.2011.09.003

Wilson, K. G., & DuFrene, T. (2009). *Mindfulness for two: An acceptance and commitment therapy approach to mindfulness in psychotherapy.* Oakland, CA: New Harbinger Publications.

Wilson, K. G., & Sandoz, E. K. (2008). Mindfulness, values, and the therapeutic relationship in acceptance and commitment therapy. In S. Hick & T. Bein (Eds.), *Mindfulness and the therapeutic relationship* (pp. 89–106). New York, NY: Guilford Press.

Wittorf, A., Wiedemann, G., Buchkremer, G., & Klingberg, S. (2007). Prediction of community outcome in schizophrenia 1 year after discharge from inpatient treatment. *European Archives of Psychiatry and Clinical Neuroscience, 258,* 48–58. doi:10.1007/s00406-007-0761-z

Wykes, T., & Reeder, C. (2005). *Cognitive remediation therapy for schizophrenia: Theory and practice.* New York, NY: Routledge / Taylor & Francis Group.

Wykes, T., Reeder, C., Huddy, V., Taylor, R., Wood, H., Ghirasim, N., et al. (2012). Developing models of how cognitive improvements change functioning: Mediation, moderation, and moderated mediation. *Schizophrenia Research, 138,* 88–93.

Young, J. E., & Brown, G. (1994). Young Schema Questionnaire (2nd ed.). In J. E. Young (Ed.), *Cognitive therapy for personality disorders: A schema-focused approach* (rev. ed., pp. 63–76). Sarasota, FL: Professional Resource Press.

Zautra, A. J., Hall, J. S., & Murray, K. E. (2010). Resilience: A new definition of health for people and communities. In J. W. Reich, A. J. Zautra, & J. S. Hall (Eds.), *Handbook of adult resilience* (pp. 3–30). New York, NY: Guilford Press.

Nicola P. Wright, PhD, CPsych, is a clinical psychologist in the schizophrenia program of the Royal Ottawa Health Care Group (The Royal). She also held the roles of chief of psychology and director of training for the Royal's Psychology Residency Program and served as president of the Canadian Council of Professional Psychology Programs. Wright provides individual and group therapy, as well as professional training workshops, integrating acceptance and commitment; mindfulness; and compassion-focused approaches in cognitive behavioral therapy (CBT) for people who experience psychosis. Wright is an active researcher and clinical professor in the School of Psychology at the University of Ottawa and a lecturer with the department of psychiatry, University of Ottawa. In addition, she is a founding member of the Canadian Association of CBT and a staff supervisor with the Beck Institute of CBT. Wright lives in Ottawa, Canada.

Douglas Turkington, MD, is a major research figure within the history of the development of cognitive behavioral therapy (CBT) for schizophrenia. He is a fellow of the Royal College of Psychiatrists and founding fellow of the Faculty of Cognitive Therapy in Philadelphia. He has written more than one hundred articles and more than half a dozen books on the subject of CBT for psychosis. Turkington lives in Newcastle, England.

Owen Kelly, PhD, CPsych, graduated from Carleton University with a specialization in behavioral neuroscience and completed a postdoctoral respecialization in clinical psychology at Fielding Graduate University. He is a clinical psychologist in private practice at the Ottawa Institute of Cognitive Behavioral Therapy. He is currently an adjunct research professor in the department of neuroscience, and lecturer in the department of psychology at Carleton University. Kelly resides in Ottawa, Canada.

Dave Davies, PhD, CPsych, received his doctorate in psychology from Queen's University in Kingston, Canada. He is a clinical psychologist and director of training at the Ottawa Institute of Cognitive Behavioral Therapy, and serves as clinical professor in the School of Psychology at the University of Ottawa, and lecturer in the department of psychiatry at the University of Ottawa. He is a founding member of the Canadian Association of Cognitive·Behavioral Therapy. Davies lives in Ottawa, Canada.

Andrew M. Jacobs, PsyD, CPsych, received his PsyD in clinical psychology from the Virginia Consortium Program in Clinical Psychology: College of William and Mary, Eastern Virginia Medical School, Norfolk State University, and Old Dominion University, and completed a postdoctoral fellowship in anxiety disorders at McMaster University/St. Joseph's Healthcare, Hamilton, Canada. He is clinical psychologist at the Royal Ottawa Health Care Group Anxiety Disorders Program, clinical professor in the School of Psychology at the University of Ottawa, and lecturer in the department of psychiatry at the University of Ottawa. Jacobs lives in Ottawa, Canada.

Jennifer Hopton, MA, is completing her PhD in clinical psychology at the University of Ottawa. Her research and clinical interests are in the areas of trauma, psychosis, substance use, community psychology, program evaluation, and mindfulness. She resides in southern Ontario, Canada.

Foreword author **Aaron T. Beck, MD**, is the president of the Beck Institute for Cognitive Behavior Therapy, and University Professor Emeritus of Psychiatry at the University of Pennsylvania. Dr. Beck developed cognitive therapy in the early 1960s as a psychiatrist at the University of Pennsylvania. He has published over 500 articles and 19 books and has lectured throughout the world. Dr. Beck is the recipient of many honors from professional and scientific organizations, including America's Nobel, the Lasker Clinical Medical Research Award.

Index

Register your **new harbinger** titles for additional benefits!

When you register your **new harbinger** title—purchased in any format, from any source—you get access to benefits like the following:

- Downloadable accessories like printable worksheets and extra content

- Instructional videos and audio files

- Information about updates, corrections, and new editions

Not every title has accessories, but we're adding new material all the time.

Access free accessories in 3 easy steps:

1. Sign in at NewHarbinger.com (or **register** to create an account).

2. Click on **register a book**. Search for your title and click the **register** button when it appears.

3. Click on the **book cover or title** to go to its details page. Click on **accessories** to view and access files.

That's all there is to it!

If you need help, visit:

NewHarbinger.com/accessories

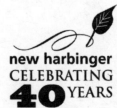

new harbinger
CELEBRATING
40 YEARS

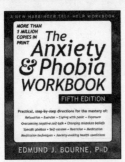
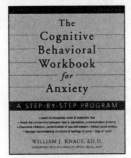
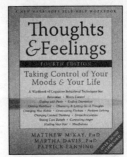
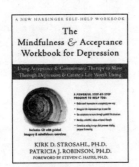
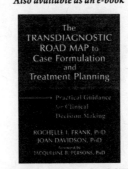
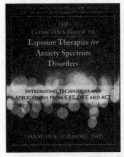

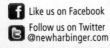